The LOW CARB WEIGHT-LOSS COOKBOOK

KATIE & GIANCARLO CALDESI

with Jenny Phillips and Dr Jen Unwin

Photography by Susan Bell

Kyle Books

This book is dedicated to Stefano Borella who has worked alongside us for more than 20 years as Pâtisserie Chef and Head Teacher at our cookery school. We have laughed, cried, cooked, eaten and drunk together and we couldn't have achieved these recipes without him.

An Hachette UK Company
www.hachette.co.uk

First published in Great Britain in 2022
by Kyle Books, an imprint of Octopus Publishing Group Limited
Carmelite House
50 Victoria Embankment
London EC4Y 0DZ

www.kylebooks.co.uk
www.octopusbooksusa.com

ISBN: 978 085783 983 1

Distributed in the US by Hachette Book Group, 1290 Avenue of the Americas,
4th and 5th Floors, New York, NY 10104

Distributed in Canada by Canadian Manda Group, 664 Annette St., Toronto, Ontario,
Canada M6S 2C8

Publisher: Joanna Copestick
Project editor: Vicky Orchard
Editorial assistants: Jenny Dye and Zakk Raja
Design: Tina Smith Hobson
Photography: Susan Bell
Food styling: Becks Wilkinson
Props styling: Hannah Wilkinson
Production: Emily Noto

A Cataloguing in Publication record for this title is available from the British Library

Printed and bound in Italy

10 9 8 7 6 5 4 3 2 1

All reasonable care has been taken in the preparation of this book but the information it contains is not intended to take the place of treatment by a qualified medical practitioner. Before making any changes in your health regime, always consult a doctor. While all the therapies detailed in this book are completely safe if done correctly, you must seek professional advice if you are in any doubt about any medical condition. Any application of the ideas and information contained in this book is at the reader's sole discretion and risk.

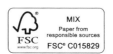

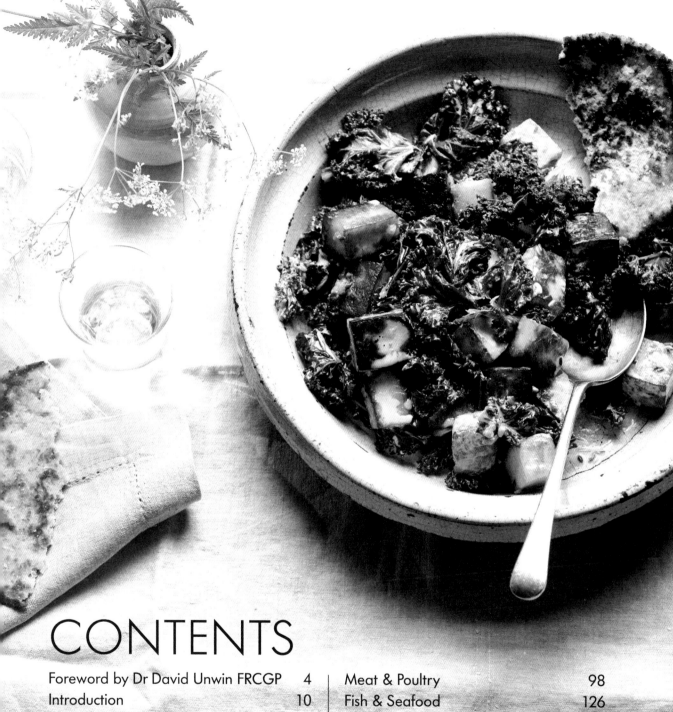

CONTENTS

FOREWORD

by Dr David Unwin FRCGP

I came out of medical school hoping to make a difference as a doctor. I had studied hard and felt well equipped to treat my future patients. My greatest efforts were to memorize the *British National Formulary* listing all the drugs at my disposal. My bible and greatest weapon against ill health, it never left my pocket. I am a slow learner, but I gradually became disappointed in the difference I was making to improve the lives of my patients. I saw antibiotics cure life-threatening infections, but by degrees I realized that the drugs I was giving were merely "sticking plasters" that didn't get to the real causes of illnesses or deliver true good health.

I remember one particular patient who was morbidly obese and on 17 different drugs, including Prozac, metformin for type 2 diabetes, and codeine. Despite all these medications, life was a real struggle for her: her knees and back still hurt, her ankles were painfully swollen, climbing stairs was incredibly hard. She struggled with low self-esteem and sleep apnoea at night. This was not good health; I began to worry I was failing many patients like this. How many drugs would she still need if I could help her lose weight, or better still not become overweight in the first place? Around the same time, I began to notice that obesity was becoming far more common, as were all the conditions associated with carrying excess weight: cardiovascular disease, hypertension, type 2 diabetes, depression and poor self-esteem, sleep apnoea, many forms of cancer, lethargy, joint pain and fatty liver disease. Across the UK, and worldwide, others were noticing the same thing.

> I believe we have eaten our way into this epidemic of obesity and diabetes, but the good news is that we can eat our way out of it.

The World Health Organization estimates that rates of obesity have tripled since I was seventeen (1975). Even worse, the number of obese young people has quadrupled, so that more than 124 million children and adolescents are affected worldwide. It's an epidemic!

To be able to help overweight patients, I needed to figure out the cause of the problem. It's often pointed out that being overweight runs in families. Does this mean it's a genetic problem, or is it just that families tend to eat the same foods? Well, hair colour is genetic, but there is no way the number of people with blond hair could triple in 45 years, yet this is exactly what has happened with obesity. Clearly something we are doing in modern life is affecting rates of obesity. This is good news because it means that the obesity epidemic is not hopeless. If we find out what the causes are, we can return to a world where obesity was so much rarer.

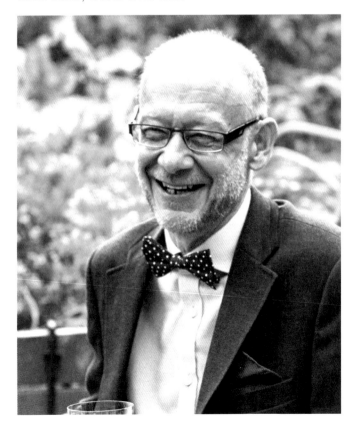

MY LOW-CARB EPIPHANY

For many years, I subscribed to the conventional view that being overweight is simply a result of calories in being greater than calories out (CICO), the surfeit being stored as fat. So, until 2012 I advised my patients to cut their calories (which often meant following a low-fat diet) and weight loss would follow. But it didn't, or not permanently. I saw so much yo-yo dieting, not least in my wife Jen, whose weight bounced up and down for decades as she starved herself for a while and then just gave up when she couldn't stand it any longer. Then one day in 2012 a patient walked in who turned all this on its head. She had lost so much weight that I didn't recognize her! When we did blood tests, we saw that she had also reversed her type 2 diabetes, but to my amazement she was still eating fat, and it was sugar and starchy carbs she had given up. My fascination with a low-carb diet started that very day and has changed my life.

My wife Jen (a clinical psychologist specializing in hope and behaviour change) and I started a low-carb group in my GP practice and, together with our practice nurse Heather, we trialled a low-carb diet. Along with 18 volunteer patients, we met every Monday night and learned about low carb together. The results were eventually published and, since then, the offer of a low-carb approach to type 2 diabetes has been taken up by hundreds of patients in our practice. Jen and I have been running our low-carb clinic for over eight years now and have published data on more than 330 people. We have seen significant improvements in so many medical conditions: blood pressure, liver function, lipid profiles, eczema, depression and heart health, our list keeps growing! The average weight loss is 10.9kg (1st 7lb). The greatest loss we have seen is 63.5kg (10 stone) in a patient who presented with sleep apnoea and was so heavy they struggled to breathe at night. Their weight-loss completely transformed their life! Many people have been able to come off prescribed medication so our practice now spends £58,000 less on drugs for diabetes per year than is average for our area. To date, over 100 of my patients have achieved drug-free

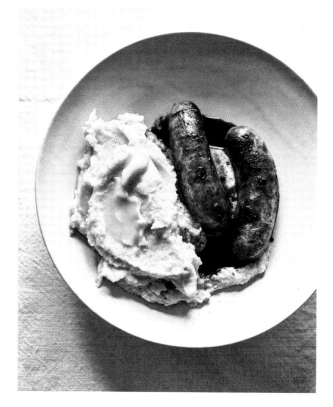

remission of their type 2 diabetes! Both Jen and I eat low carb to this day, not only because we enjoy the food so much but also because of the health benefits. My blood pressure is much improved and I need 1½ hours less sleep a day. Jen is about 12.7kg (2 stone) lighter and has far fewer migraines and less joint pain.

WHAT IS A LOW-CARB DIET?

So, what do we mean by low carb? While cutting out sugar and starchy carbs, a low-carb diet focuses on healthy protein and fats like meat, fish, eggs, dairy and nuts alongside a rainbow of vegetables and berries. A low-carb diet contains less than 130g carbs per day (the average western diet contains around 250g carbs a day). You can vary the amount of carbs you consume according to our CarbScale (see page 24) and your personal health goals. But as Jenny Phillips explains on pages 14–19, going low carb isn't as simple as just cutting out the sugar you put in your tea and coffee. Sugar is everywhere! Basically, there are three sources:

❋ **Naturally sugary foods** like honey, raisins or fruit juice.
❋ **Foods with added sugars** like biscuits, cakes and jam.
❋ **Starchy carbohydrate foods** that digest down into sugar; bread, rice, breakfast cereals or potatoes are potent sources of sugar.

A CALORIE IS JUST A CALORIE *Isn't it?*

Central to the calories-in-calories-out (CICO) model of weight gain is the idea that all calories are equal. But compare how you feel after eating 400 calories of salmon (300g/10½oz) to 400 calories of biscuits (about five biscuits). Most of us would see that as a big helping of salmon and, alongside some salad or greens, makes a meal that leaves us full, but we'd consider a few biscuits as "only a snack". I would still want my dinner! So, you can see how different foods affect appetite differently, and that hunger is dependent on the source of the calories we consume.

LOW-CARB *for* WEIGHT-LOSS

Over time, eating too much sugar, and starchy carbs that digest down into sugar, can increase your appetite, cause weight gain and even increase your blood pressure. When your blood sugar increases from consuming sugar or starchy carbs, the pancreas gland produces the hormone insulin to lower it again. It does this by pushing sugar out of the blood into different types of cells. Some is pushed into muscle cells for energy, but if you consume more sugar than you need for exercise, the excess is pushed into your belly or liver cells, where it is turned into fat. In fact, that is how most of us got our middle-aged spread! So, a sugary snack of biscuits will do several things. Initially your blood sugar will increase (giving some people that "sugar rush" that Jen explains on page 34), but this stimulates the pancreas to produce insulin, which brings your blood sugar rapidly down, so you feel hungry again and go back to the cookie jar. I call this the sugar cycle. Unfortunately, if you are on the sugar cycle it can lead to chronically raised insulin levels, which is known as hyperinsulinemia and is linked to a surprisingly large number of modern illnesses, such as cancer (particularly breast and colorectal cancer), inflammation, fatty liver disease, dementia, infertility, type 2 diabetes, hypertension and heart disease.

Hunger

Low blood sugar   Sugar cycle   Dietary sugar

Insulin   High blood sugar

Insulin can also be seen as a "fat fertilizer", increasing hunger and turning sugar into fat, an obvious cause of being overweight. A high-sugar, high-insulin diet also causes your kidneys to hoard salt and water, tending to increase blood pressure and cause bloating. Over time, insulin causes fat to build up in the liver and the pancreas itself, so firstly your insulin doesn't work as well, and secondly the pancreas struggles to produce insulin (as it's full of fat). This means it is difficult to keep your blood sugar at a healthy level and you may well develop type 2 diabetes. Over time, higher blood sugars damage the lining of your arteries, leading to many of the heart and circulatory problems associated with diabetes.

Surely we need some carbs? Don't we? Well, the short answer is no. We are a dual-fuel engine, able to burn either sugar or fat for energy. There are vital proteins and fats but no vital carbohydrates. In fact, in an emergency your body can make sugar out of fat or protein, which is called gluconeogenesis. (There is an important exception to this rule: some people on prescribed medication, particularly for diabetes, might have a problem with

Over time, higher blood sugars damage the lining of your arteries, leading to many of the heart and circulatory problems associated with diabetes.

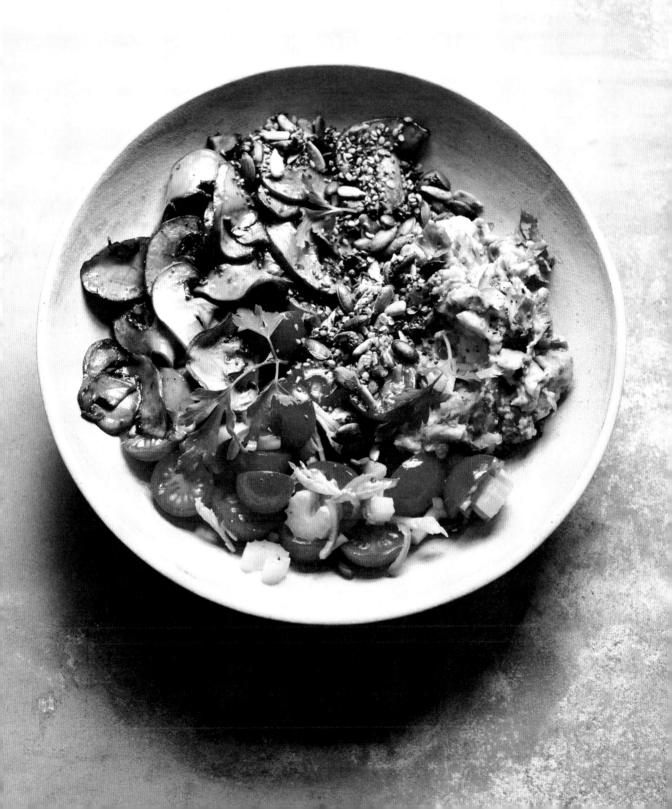

a low-carb diet and should ask their doctor before embarking on major dietary changes.)

Many of you will have heard people blame their weight on a slow metabolism. So, what is your metabolism? It's how food is converted into energy and how that energy is used for thinking, moving and growth. The more calories used up by your metabolism, the more weight you will lose! Here too, we find that different foods affect your metabolism differently. Studies have shown that sugar and starchy foods actually slow your metabolism, making weight gain more likely.

BECOMING A FAT-BURNER

Many of my patients are really interested in becoming a fat-burner because fat is what they want to get rid of. A related question is: why are overweight people hungry anyway? They have kilos of fat reserves that could deliver 9 calories per gram. I was hungry all day, every day, until I was 55 years old, despite my growing middle-aged spread. Again, insulin is part of the riddle. Insulin wants you to burn sugar preferentially to fat, so it actually blocks your ability to burn fat. Eating just a few biscuits throughout the day will keep your insulin high enough to stop you burning your own fat reserves, adding to your hunger. The thing that most surprises my low-carb patients when they change their diets is that they are not hungry any more.

HOW LOW TO GO *and the keto diet*

I mentioned earlier that a low-carb diet is one containing less than 130g carbohydrates. But should it be 100g, 30g or 10g carbs? There is a spectrum of low-carb diets all the way from just lower carb to strict keto. Jenny Phillips explains more on pages 14–19, but one of the issues to bear in mind is how much fat you are hoping to burn. The negative effect that insulin has on fat burning only diminishes slightly if you reduce your carbs to 50g per day. If you cut your carbs to less than 50g a day, then you will start burning far more fat, so much so that you produce ketones, a by-product of fat burning. This is the basis of the keto diet where ketones can be found in the blood or urine. The keto diet has increased in global popularity over the past few years and though some healthcare professionals worry it is extreme, there are many who are cautiously optimistic. Certainly, Jen and I have been in ketosis for most of the past eight years, and so far, so good! The main advantage for me is mental clarity, as I feel my brain works better. For Jen, it is the only way she can keep her weight steady and avoid food cravings.

SNACKING *and listening to your body*

It is possible that the more often you eat, the hungrier you are. This potentially makes weight loss on a "little and often" diet difficult. In particular, I find snacking makes weight loss far less likely. Sadly, for years I told my patients that "breakfast is the most important meal of the day" without a shred of evidence, and even forced myself to eat it though I wasn't hungry. In general, if you are overweight and not hungry, why eat? I gave up breakfast years ago and then read a paper in *The British Medical Journal* concluding: "Caution is needed when recommending breakfast for weight loss in adults, as it could have the opposite effect."

I used to be in the habit of eating a few cookies with each tea or coffee throughout my working day. We kept the cookie jar by the kettle at the practice. Psychological factors are clearly important in how much we eat and when. For some people, even stronger psychological factors are at play in eating behaviour. Jen and I

Eating just a few biscuits throughout the day will keep your insulin high enough to stop you burning your own fat reserves.

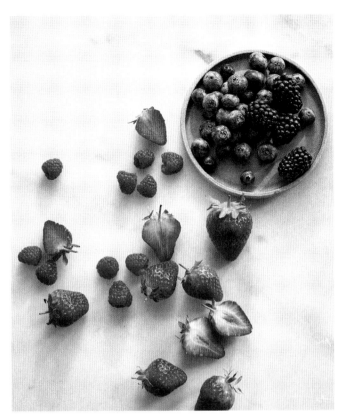

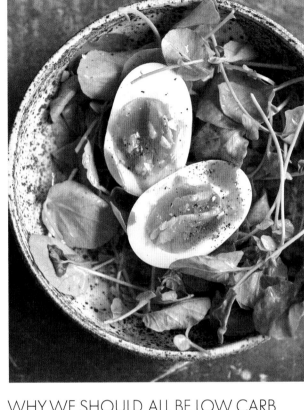

believe sugar addiction is something that many of us struggle with. Jen will discuss some tips to help tackle this on page 35, but related to this is the effect of junk or ultra-processed foods, designed to be hyperpalatable and difficult to resist. There is some evidence that these foods are linked with an increased all-cause mortality; for example, a study was conducted on over 222,000 people participating in the Moli-sani Project. By analyzing their eating habits and following their health conditions for over eight years, researchers noticed that those consuming a high amount of ultra-processed foods had an increased risk of death, not just from cardiovascular disease but from any cause. The main culprit could be sugar, which in ultra-processed foods is added in substantial amounts. But the answer seems more complex. "According to our analyses", explains Dr Augusto Di Castelnuovo, "the excess of sugar does play a role, but it accounts only for 40 per cent of the increased death risk. Our idea is that an important part is played by industrial processing itself, able to induce deep modifications in the structure and composition of nutrients."

WHY WE SHOULD ALL BE LOW CARB

So cutting junk food is a good idea for everyone but what about going low carb? In my practice we have seen weight loss, improvements in blood pressure and liver function, greater mental clarity and, of course, drug-free remission of type 2 diabetes. Perhaps you don't currently have any of these problems, many young people don't. But could a poor diet lead to these conditions in the future? Why not sort your diet before you are ill? Certainly, I wish I had understood the benefits of lifestyle medicine over lifelong medication much earlier in my medical career.

See yourself as an experiment, as Jen says (see pages 34–35), notice what works for you and do more of it. This book is part of your journey towards delicious food that helps reduce hunger and optimize your metabolism. We want to share our low-carb enthusiasm and what we have learned to help you enjoy healthy, nutritionally dense, tasty food every day to lose weight and maintain a healthy weight for life. If you get that right, you will lose weight and enjoy yourself into the bargain, as I and so many of my patients have done.

Good luck!

Follow me on Twitter @lowcarbGP

LOSING WEIGHT FOR LIFE
Katie & Giancarlo

We started this journey as a family around nine years ago with a month of giving up any food that wasn't "natural". Our youngest son Flavio was ten years old at the time, which made Giancarlo think back to when he was the same age, growing up on a rural smallholding in Tuscany. Giancarlo was fit and lean at that age; he would never have had junk food (like our children at that time) and enjoyed a varied diet and home-cooked food. There were a few times that he went to bed hungry, as money was scarce, but generally life was good, he was happy and rarely ill. He and his family lived off the land, totally in sync with the seasons. After an evening spent comparing his and Flavio's young lives, we decided to make the change.

Our new way of eating was going to be based on the cooking from the traditional country kitchens of Italy: la cucina povera. Literally translated as the "kitchen of the poor" but ironically anything but poor-quality nutrition. From that day on, if it came in a packet, we weren't going to eat it. Out went the large bags of crisps, the sliced white bread, the sugary cereals, the sweets, chocolate spread and cookies and plenty more. I hadn't wanted a showdown with the kids so as I took away their familiar foods, I replaced them with other tempting, natural alternatives. The crisps turned into roasted walnuts and pecans, the chocolate spread on white bread became cubes of cheese and apple, and the boys never even noticed!

What we did notice was how we felt – we all lost weight and really enjoyed the month. We used the car less, went for family walks rather than sat glued to the TV, we bought chickens for the garden, planted seeds, learned from a professional how to light a fire and cook over it in the woods, we bought pheasants and discovered how to pluck and butcher them. We were back in touch with real food and loved every minute of it. We never did go back to our lives of crisps and cheap chocolate bars but Giancarlo was still eating bread, pasta, rice and potatoes by the score. They were still natural in our minds but we hadn't gone far enough.

Then Giancarlo was told by his doctor that he had type 2 diabetes and by nutritionist Jenny Phillips that he was highly gluten-intolerant. He was devastated. He gave up gluten, and Jenny suggested that we tried a low-carb diet to combat his diabetes.

I wanted to make Giancarlo better and I knew weight-loss was essential, so we started eating low carb. Giancarlo is now nearly 4 stone lighter and I am pleased to say he will soon be looking forward to entering his eighth year of remission from type 2 diabetes. I am a size 12 instead of size 14 to 16, which I was for about ten years. Low carb is now a way of life; it has helped us to lose weight and keep that weight off. We are both less tired, have more energy, we can exercise harder and feel we have better immune systems. Giancarlo no longer suffers with arthritis (this could be the gluten-free side of his diet), his psoriasis has improved, the eyesight in his left eye is better, he has more feeling in his feet, he sleeps better, has got rid of his sleep apnoea and can tie his own shoelaces once more. Read more about our low-carb lifestyle at www.thegoodkitchentable.com.

> Low carb is now a way of life; it has helped us to lose weight and keep that weight off. We are both less tired, have more energy, we can exercise harder and feel we have better immune systems.

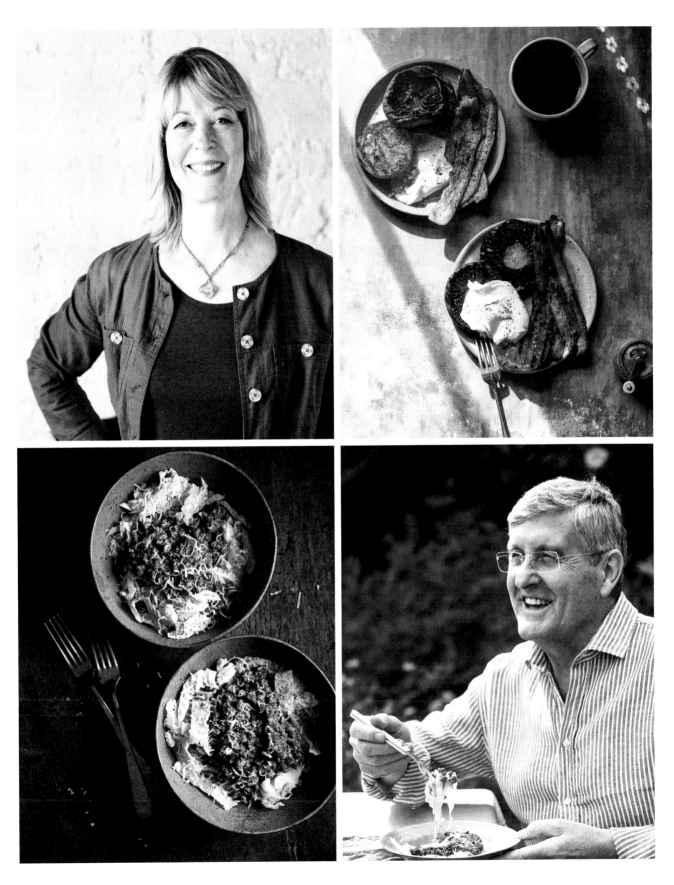

Giancarlo has to be stricter than me to keep his type 2 diabetes in remission, so he tends to eat twice a day and keep his carbs under 30–50g net carbs a day. I can consume 50–75g net carbs a day. Any blips in our weight management can be repaired in a few days. Our sons, Giorgio and Flavio, are on 75–100g net carbs a day, so you can see how you can flex your carbs according to your age, health and body type (see more on the CarbScale on page 24).

In essence, we keep our daily carb count low, enjoy good fats and eat a good portion of protein at most meals, as we know this keeps us going until the next one. What I want to shout out is to use as many different vegetables as possible! They are good for your body, gut health and digestion and bulk out a meal without resorting to starchy carbs. The goal is to switch your metabolism from storing fat to burning fat as an efficient energy source, as Dr David Unwin explains on page 8. We are low-carb not no-carb, and since we run Italian restaurants and love our own food, we do enjoy the occasional bowl of fresh pasta or a slice of pizza, but it is a rarity not a daily occurrence. We always make sure there are low-carb options for our customers and ourselves so that everyone can eat this way.

MAKE TIME *to* MOVE

When Giancarlo and I remember our mothers, they were always on the move, walking through the fields, cycling into town, running up and down stairs and doing the housework. Hardly anything was automated, no vacuum cleaners, no remote controls. Now you have to really make the effort to move. Although weight-loss is largely won in the kitchen, it doesn't hurt to add a little more exercise into your day. Kwame Richardson, personal trainer, shares his advice:

As a personal trainer I have had the joys of not only seeing clients experience fat loss and improved fitness but, just as importantly, improvement in their mental state. It is well known that moving more increases the release of endorphins which help to boost your mood. For that reason alone, why wouldn't you want to move more?

Choose an activity that you enjoy – Being active doesn't have to involve running or lifting heavy weights. It could involve walking, cycling, swimming or even dancing. Whatever you do, just move. You may feel at the start that it is an effort, but as those endorphins are released and you experience the feel-good factor, you'll find yourself looking forward to it.

Start slowly – Always start at a comfortable level. It is tempting to be overly ambitious in trying to reach an end goal, but in doing so you are likely to overwork yourself, leading to mental burnout or potential injury. Try starting with just 10 minutes of a particular activity daily and build from there.

Set realistic goals – While you may have visions of a flat stomach or bulging biceps, it is important to know that these are not achieved overnight. Set shorter goals that can be attained. For example, if you are walking for 10 minutes three days a week, try and increase the length of time by 10 per cent each week. You will find this rewarding and enjoyable. Ideally, you should work towards meeting the government guidelines of 150 minutes of moderate exercise along with an all-over body weights routine two days a week. This may seem like a lot but when spread over seven days it works out around 22 minutes each day.

Consistency – In your quest to become active aim to be consistent. Choose a time of day that you can dedicate to exercise and stick to it. Doing this will get you on the path to a happy and healthier lifestyle.

Our TOP 10 LOW-CARB tips

1 Understand the logic behind this lifestyle. Know your carbs, which to have and which to avoid. Only eat food that you recognize. Read the label, visualize the ingredients and ask yourself whether they are low carb or not (see page 36). If you don't know what an ingredient looks like, don't eat it.

2 Don't eat ultra-processed food such as ready meals, drinks in cans or fast-food takeaways – the available calories are usually high due to processing. Sugar is added to 80 per cent of supermarket foods. Instead get organized and cook at home or go to restaurants where the food is cooked fresh and be wise with your order.

3 Avoid putting yourself in the position of having to eat a sandwich or other carby snack. Be prepared and take low-carb food wherever you go or make sure you can get it easily.

4 Do not snack between meals. If you want an ultralight meal because you aren't very hungry, then that is fine, but enjoy it instead of a meal not as well as one. (See page 36.)

5 Keep a food diary. We are so good at kidding ourselves, that the only way to really know what and how much you are eating is to commit to recording everything that passes your lips! You can do this simply by photographing everything you eat and drink on your phone or by writing it down.

6 Eat enough protein at every meal. Whenever I don't have enough, I end up picking between meals. I often have three eggs at one meal, cooked chicken livers, a whole can of sardines, a steak or chicken breast, so I feel properly full and then I can forget about food between meals (apart from the fact that I am surrounded by it and usually writing about it!).

7 Choose your treats wisely. We are naturally hedonists and, as restaurateurs, temptation is everywhere; we are in the business of indulgence. To cope with this, Giancarlo enjoys a treat every other day; this might be a small low-carb dessert that I keep in the fridge for him, a glass of dry fizz or a bowl of yogurt, berries and nuts with 1 teaspoon of honey. He hates to feel imprisoned by a "diet"; this way he feels free and is still low carb. I like a small glass of red wine in the evenings with one square of 90% dark chocolate.

8 Notice how you look and feel. Giancarlo can feel his eyes hurt if he eats too much sugar the day before. I feel tired and bloated if I have indulged in carbs or don't include enough vegetables in my meals. This helps you understand which foods suit your body.

9 If you feel peckish, have a glass of water; it helps perk you up as well as fill you up. Sometimes you think you are hungry when actually you are simply thirsty.

10 Remember it is the foods you leave out as well as what you choose to eat. Make a rule for yourself never to have a second helping, to walk away from the cookie jar and make a cup of tea instead – it will all add up to helping you reach your weight-loss goals by the end of the week.

THE LOW-CARB LOWDOWN

A tried and tested way of eating for health and weight loss

Jenny Phillips, nutritionist

www.InspiredNutrition.co.uk

My own journey to low-carb eating was born out of a cancer diagnosis in my late thirties. Fortunately, I made a full recovery following medical treatment, but I really wanted to ensure I optimized my chances of a long and healthy life. I was amazed to learn how food could interact with your metabolism, for better or for worse. For me, my change of diet meant I lost weight naturally, my sleep improved and my energy levels soared. Nearly 20 years on from my diagnosis, I feel fitter and healthier than I did in my thirties! I no longer need to take any medications, which I previously used to manage asthma, hay fever, indigestion and debilitating period pains. This experience led to a fascination with diet and nutrition, and I qualified with a degree in nutritional medicine and as a yoga teacher in 2010. I now specialize in helping clients to improve their health and achieve their weight goals through nutrition and lifestyle coaching – alongside their medical treatment if they have a diagnosed condition. This is how I met the Caldesis, working with Giancarlo to help reverse his type 2 diabetes, improve his health and lose weight. That all three can be achieved by changing to a low-carb diet is nothing short of amazing.

Every day I see people like Giancarlo transform their health when they embrace a low-carb way of eating. Most telling is that if they do take a short break and introduce more carby treats, for a few weeks over Christmas or a holiday perhaps, they tell me they can't wait to get back to their low-carb "diet" because they feel so much better on it!

Common reasons why people seek my help are digestive issues, hormonal imbalances (like menopause), general fatigue or support for more complex health conditions. But weight-loss is the most prevalent health goal, I think because obesity has become so widespread and has such a significant impact on all aspects of health.

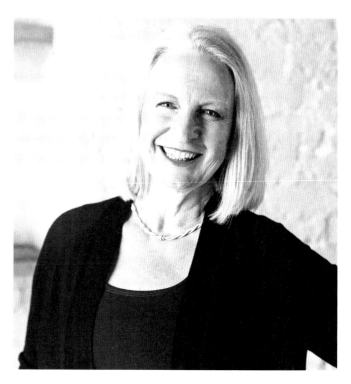

It is typical to lose around half a stone in the first three weeks of moving to our weight-loss plan, alongside many other positive side effects, including **feeling liberated** from food cravings; **enjoying better energy** and sleep; and **improved digestion**, particularly issues like acid reflux, and **feeling more in control**.

Over the past 11 years, I have found that low carb is the most universal and effective way to eat well. It is just going back to enjoying simple ingredients that make tasty meals and spending some time in the kitchen. Low carb can be tweaked to meet specific dietary requirements, whether for vegetarians, carnivores, or those following the popular paleo or keto diets. You can exclude any foods that don't suit you and embrace a wide range of ingredients that your body will love.

Challenging CONVENTIONAL DIETS

The chances are that you've come to this book because you've tried a range of diets and have yet to find a way of eating that helps you lose weight and keep it off. Yes, massively restricting how much you eat can and does result in a shift on the scales, but all too often you find that your weight rebounds. Or maybe you feel that you are always on a diet, making sacrifices in your food choices and taking the joy out of eating?

You may also be confused by the myriad of often conflicting messages around healthy eating. Official health advice for weight loss is based on creating a calorie deficit – you are told to "eat less and move more". This may sound intuitively sensible – until you start to unpick what it really means.

Food contains three macronutrients: fats, carbs and protein (see page 17 for more detail). If you are creating a "low-calorie meal", you will avoid fat, simply because it contains more calories than carbs or protein: fat contains 9 calories per gram while carbs and protein contain 4 calories per gram. The result is the "Eatwell plate" and current health guidelines which advise you to "base your meals on starchy carbs", such as bread, cereals, pasta, rice and potatoes. The trouble is that these foods break down very quickly into glucose, a type of sugar, disrupting your blood sugar levels and potentially leading to weight gain, pre-diabetes or even type 2 diabetes.

A good example of this is the popular rice cake, which is often eaten as a quick snack by people aiming to eat well and lose weight. Two are just 52 calories, but with 11.2g carbs, or the equivalent of more than 2 teaspoons of sugar! Now as your bloodstream can only carry 1 teaspoon of sugar at any one time, this is likely to cause blood sugar swings.

On the other hand, foods with a higher fat and protein content are more satisfying; they don't disrupt your blood sugar levels and they help to fill you up. No more cravings or obsessing about food, but the quiet confidence of feeling your appetite is under control. Consequently, most people following a low-carb diet

Melanie's story
LOW CARB AS A PESCATARIAN

As the manager of a busy kindergarten, Melanie is on her feet all day. She recently found out about low carb through Jenny's nutrition reset programme and was shocked to discover that her previous eating habits, which she thought were very healthy, needed tweaking to help her lose weight and improve her health.

"Before joining the low-carb group, I thought that I was doing really well with healthy eating. I ticked all the main boxes – eating at least five fruit and veg a day, hardly having any alcohol, fasting by skipping breakfast and eating low-fat foods, especially rice cakes and baked potatoes. I felt proud that I was taking veggie soup and three pieces of fruit for lunch, and always had a healthy supper. But the bit that I just couldn't control was coming home from work and having a mini binge in the kitchen while cooking dinner. I'd start with more low-fat rice cakes, but quickly sweep into jam sandwiches and other sweet things. I assumed it was my lack of willpower that caused me to feel I constantly had to be on a diet.

As a pescatarian, the first thing I learned was that I was not eating enough protein and so I made a big shift to increase eggs, fish, nuts and dairy products in my diet. I cut down on fruit and still enjoyed lots of vegetables. I experimented with low-carb breads and crackers and banished low-fat foods from my kitchen.

The changes that I felt were quick to appear. Firstly, I regained control of my teatime eating. I could plan a low-carb snack, like cheese on low-carb crackers or an egg, as I was only having two main meals a day. Rather than turning to more food, I felt satisfied, in part because I was now always having protein with my lunch. In terms of weight, I have dropped two dress sizes and lost 5cm (2in) from my waist.

But the bigger changes have been in how I feel. I am now full of energy; I walk the dog and feel like a gazelle in the woods! I used to have restless legs syndrome, which hurt and disturbed my sleep. That has completely gone. My skin, hair and sleep are so much better. My whole life feels better, and I feel so much more confident. I love the way I eat now. With cheese, cream and butter on the menu, what's not to like?"

How starchy carbs affect your blood sugar levels

Food group	Food item	Carbs	Teaspoons of sugar equivalent
Starchy foods	Basmati rice, 150g	40g	10.1
	Potato, white, 150g	26g	9.1
	French fries, 150g	32g	7.5
	Spaghetti, white, 180g	46g	6.6
	Oats, 30g	19g	4.4
	Brown bread, 30g	12g	3.3
Vegetables	Sweetcorn, 80g	18g	4
	Frozen peas, 80g	7g	1.3
	Broccoli, 80g	4g	0.2
Fruit	Banana, 120g	26g	5.9
	Apple, 120g	15g	2.2
Eggs	Eggs, 60g	0g	0

have no desire to snack between meals, thus making a significant calorie saving throughout the day.

HOW MUCH SUGAR?!

The concept of sugar equivalents has been pioneered by Dr David Unwin and is now widely used by many forward-thinking GPs and doctors. His infographics provide a visual snapshot which can instantly help people to understand why a diet based on starchy carbs can be a real problem if you are looking to improve your health or lose weight. When you consider that a portion of rice can have a similar effect on your blood sugar as eating 10 teaspoons of sugar, then you may well be quite shocked!

If you currently eat a lot of these starchy foods, you may wonder how you are going to manage such a change to your diet. Relax, you are in good hands. Katie has perfected the art of low-carb cooking, and her delicious recipes will inspire you to make changes – look forward to a slimmer, healthier and more confident you!

LOW CARB IN A NUTSHELL

As the name implies, a low-carb diet is low in sugar and starchy carbohydrate foods. So, what are these foods and how can they help you lose weight?

Carbs, or carbohydrates, are one of the three macronutrients which make up our food, along with fat and protein. Carbs contain stored energy as simple sugars; when you eat sweet or carby foods, these sugars are broken down into their most basic form – glucose – which can be used to fuel the cells in your body.

No one is in any doubt that eating lots of sweet foods like chocolate, confectionery, cookies, cakes and fizzy drinks can cause rapid weight gain. The trouble is that many of our best-loved carby foods also break down to provide way more sugar than your body can handle. Typical examples include bread, pasta, pastries, pizza, breakfast cereals, crackers, oats and rice. Blood sugar levels (also called blood glucose levels) consequently rise when they are eaten. For some people this is not an issue, and their metabolisms can cope with these surges of blood sugar. But for many of us, these surges are problematic and can lead both to weight gain and, if this style of eating continues, to issues with blood sugar regulation, potentially leading to type 2 diabetes.

When you eat more carbs than your body can manage, it does something clever to maintain your blood sugar within safe levels. Your pancreas triggers a secretion of insulin, which moves sugar out of your bloodstream and into your cells. Then it replenishes your storage system for carbs, which is called glycogen (about 2,000 calories can be stored in both the muscles and liver). Then, and this is where the weight gain kicks in, excess carbs are converted to saturated fat and stored, often around your middle, creating a "muffin top" or what some see as the start of middle-aged spread.

How STARCHY FOODS CAUSE WEIGHT GAIN

If you are the sort of person that puts on weight easily, then the chances are that you are "carbohydrate intolerant". Rather than using the sugar from carbs to fuel you and increase your energy, you are shunting it into storage as fat. Consequently, not only is your weight increasing, but you are also suffering from energy swings and possibly periods of feeling "hangry" where you feel hungry, tired and maybe even a bit angry.

Two things happen when your blood sugar levels drop, courtesy of the hormone insulin:

1. You feel really hungry. Those hangry feelings want satisfying and only more food will do. Carby eaters often graze their way through the day, consuming more calories than if they naturally controlled their blood sugar.

2. Insulin switches your body into fat-storage mode, and subsequently prevents you burning calories which you have previously stored as fat.

FAT AS FUEL

The second of the macronutrients, fat, has dual roles in your body. It is used structurally in cell membranes, your brain and nervous system and some hormones, for example cortisol and sex hormones. But, most importantly, it is also a source of stored energy – it is fuel. You are a hybrid engine and can gain your energy requirements from carbs or fat, or a combination of both.

Now, it may seem counterintuitive that if you are prone to weight gain you should consider switching to consuming more calories from fat, but bear with me. The main anti-fat story is based on the fact that fat contains more calories per gram than carbs or protein (9kcal vs 4kcal respectively). Hence the logic went: just cut out those high-calorie fatty foods and you'll lose weight. But that's not what happens. That's why you're here.

So, let's think about things a bit more carefully. What does it mean to lose weight? Where will that weight go? To achieve weight loss, you actually want to burn the calories

Mandy & David's story FREEDOM FROM SUGAR SWINGS

Mandy and her husband David share a love of good food. In the past they have followed various slimming clubs to lose weight but made a decision to try low carb after discovering *The Diabetes Weight-loss Cookbook*.

"What we really love about this new way of eating is how easy it is to follow and how flexible it is. Previously we were constantly thinking about food and counting points or calories. Our meals always included what we then thought of as 'healthy carbs' – brown rice or wholewheat pasta or bread. I could lose weight by being really strict, but I couldn't maintain it and would see my weight rebound. This meant we spent a lot of time dieting and feeling deprived.

The big difference with our low-carb menu is that I feel liberated. It was no problem giving up most of the starchy carbs and I really don't miss them. The only one I've kept is a slice of rye bread with eggs for my breakfast. We now enjoy three meals a day without spiking our blood sugar levels, which means that we don't feel hungry during the day. In fact, Jenny was quite surprised at how much I was able to eat and still consistently lose weight each week.

David also likes to cook; we plan our meals together and have got into the habit of a main weekly shop, so that we always have the ingredients we need. Planning is a real advantage when so much of our cooking is from scratch. We often make meals from the Caldesi cookbooks and they are just delicious. We also found it no problem to enjoy dinner parties and still follow the low-carb principles, including a pudding with cream!

We have both lost significant weight – David is down 4 stone and I have lost over a stone to achieve my goal of just over 10½ stone. We both feel more like exercising and our energy levels have increased. But the best thing is how easy it is to maintain, which is something I've never been able to manage before. I'm a schoolteacher and recently over half-term, I went into a maintenance phase and added a few controlled treats in addition to my low-carb meals. I was able to carry on without fretting and keep my weight within a 2lb window which I now know how to manage. I've got the tools now and have enjoyed learning about the science of low carb."

that are stored around your midriff and elsewhere as fuel. I'll say that again. The energy that is stored as fat in your body needs to be liberated and used to make energy in your cells, instead of or in addition to using the food that you eat. Bingo! Now all you need to do is work out how to encourage those fat stores to be released.

The most significant factor in your ability to consistently burn fat as fuel is the level of insulin in your blood. Insulin is a fat-storage hormone, converting excess carbs to fat stores and hindering your body's ability to release and burn its own fat stores. Because eating fat does not raise your insulin levels, you are able to switch easily between burning the calories you eat and calories you have previously stored. Eating higher-fat foods can prime your body to burn fat easily, whereas carbs (which stimulate insulin) can hinder it. The beauty of accessing your fat stores for energy is twofold: you start to shift those pesky pounds, but even more importantly, you do not feel hungry – and so you eat less. This is the secret of successful weight loss.

The IMPORTANCE OF GOOD-QUALITY PROTEIN

The third cornerstone of a low-carb diet is eating sufficient protein with every meal. Protein builds healthy, strong bodies, supports growth and repair and is essential for long-term good health.

Protein foods also help you to feel fuller for longer. A study in the Netherlands found that increasing your protein intake by 50 per cent above the minimum recommended levels had a positive effect on body composition and also on blood pressure. When protein intake was low, weight regain was more likely. In practice, I find that people often benefit from increasing their protein intake, as often they are just not eating enough. Good sources are meat, fish, eggs, dairy, nuts, seeds, pulses and vegetarian protein like soy (see table opposite).

Try to aim for 60–80g (2¼–2¾oz) protein per day, more if you have a larger frame or are very active. Do note that protein content varies significantly between foods and this chart is helpful in understanding where protein comes from:

PROTEIN CONTENT OF COMMON FOODS

High protein foods	Protein
100g (3½oz) turkey or chicken breast	35g
100g (3½oz) lean sirloin steak	34g
100g (3½oz) lamb's liver	30g
100g (3½oz) lean lamb steak	28g
100g (3½oz) Cheddar cheese	26g
100g (3½oz) pork chop	24g
100g (3½oz) cod or haddock	24g
100g (3½oz) halloumi	24g
100g (3½oz) salmon steak	23g
100g (3½oz) goat's cheese	22g
100g (3½oz) canned sardines, drained	22g
2 high-meat-content sausages (117g/4oz)	21g
Medium protein foods	
2 medium eggs (58g/2¼oz each)	16g
100g (3½oz) feta cheese	16g
100g (3½oz) peeled prawns	14g
100g (3½oz) tofu	12.6g
100g (3½oz) lentils	10.6g
Lower protein foods	
100g (3½oz) cottage cheese	7.2g
100g (3½oz) chickpeas	7.2g
100g (3½oz) full-fat Greek yogurt	5.6g
Nuts and seeds	
30g (1oz) hemp seeds	11g
30g (1oz) pumpkin seeds	8.6g
30g (1oz) sunflower seeds	7g
30g (1oz) flaxseed	6.6g
30g (1oz) whole almonds	6g
30g (1oz) chia seeds	5.5g

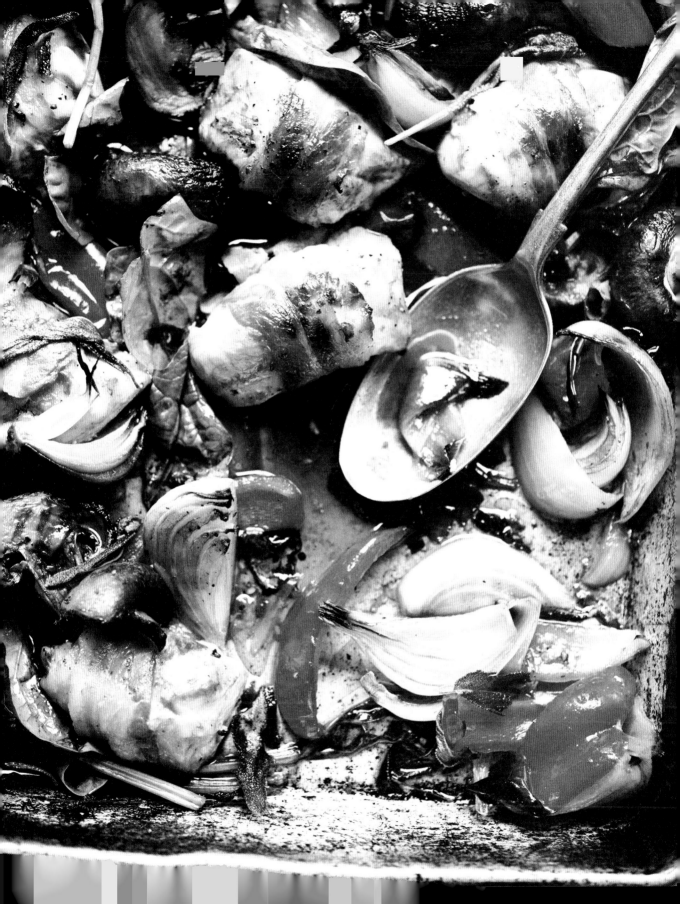

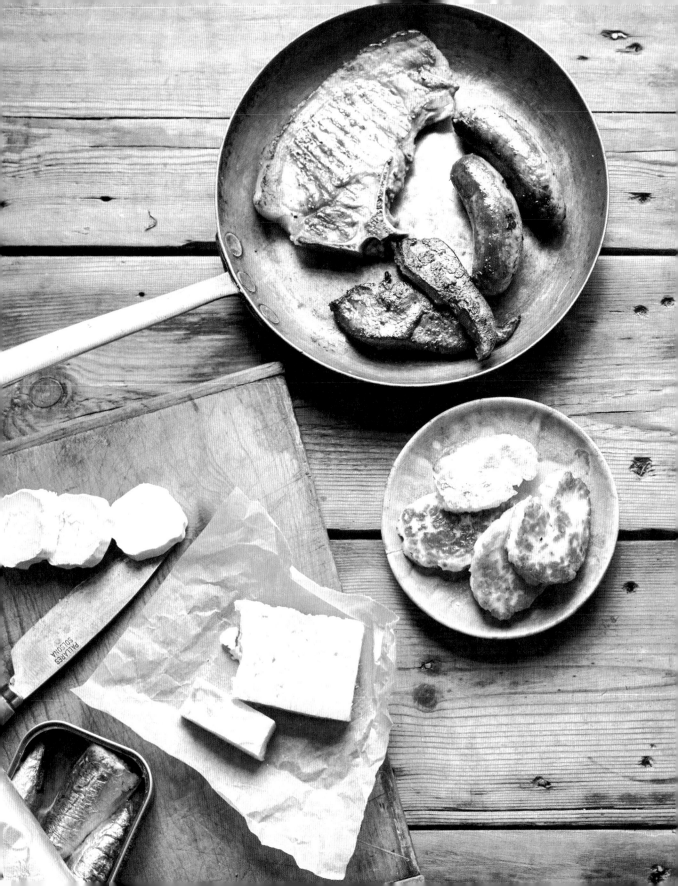

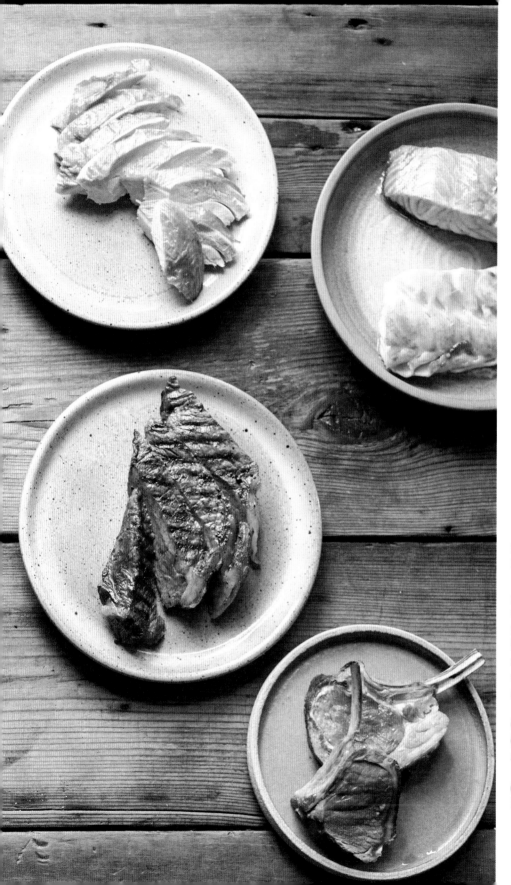

High protein foods

Pork chop (24g/per 100g); lamb's liver (30g/per 100g); 2 high-meat-content sausages (21g/per 117g); chicken breast (35g/per 100g); salmon steak (23g/per 100g); cod (24g/per 100g); goat's cheese (22g/per 100g); Cheddar cheese (26g/per 100g); halloumi (24g/per 100g); lean sirloin steak (34g/per 100g); canned sardines (22g/per 100g); lean lamb steak (28g/per 100g).

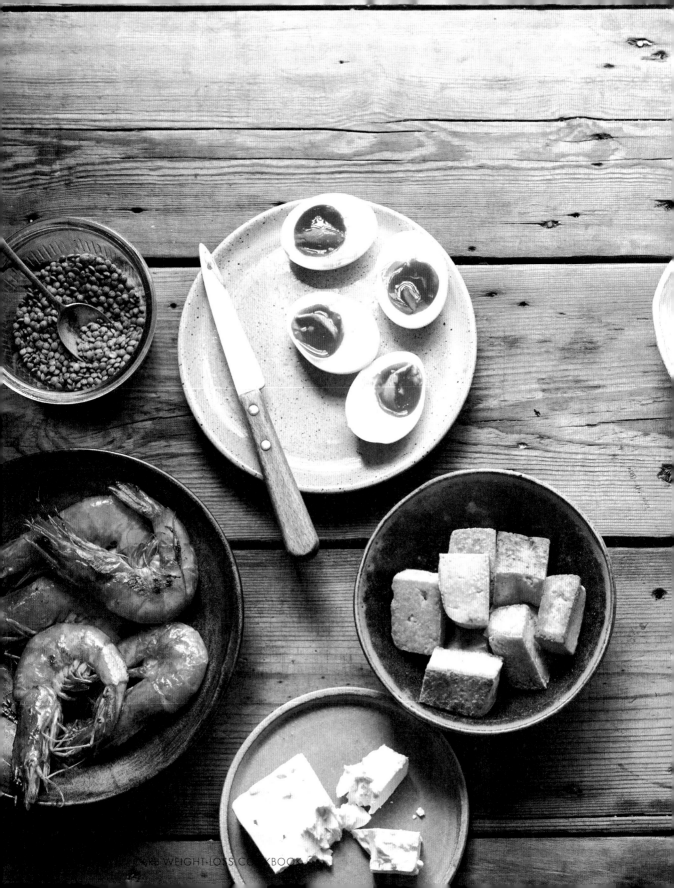

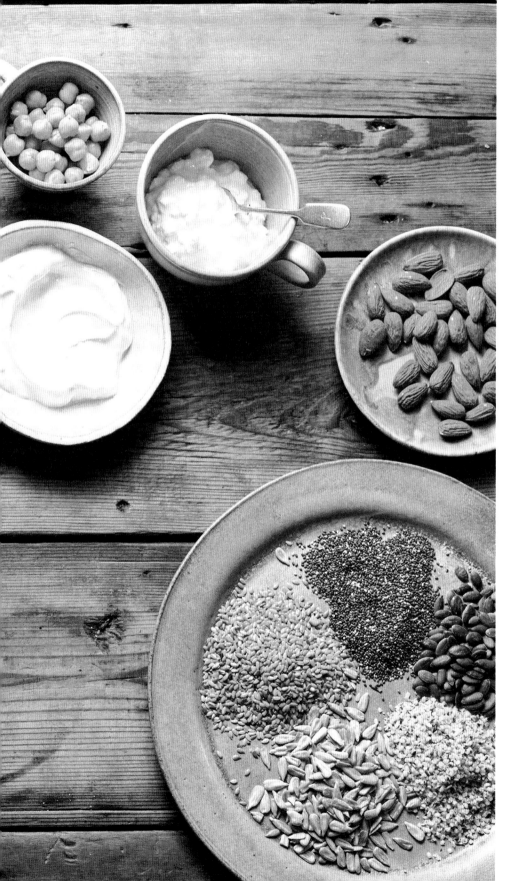

Medium–lower protein foods

Lentils (10.6g/per 100g); 2 medium eggs (16g/per 58g); chickpeas (7.2g/per 100g); full-fat Greek yogurt (5.6g/per 100g); cottage cheese (7.2g/per 100g); whole almonds (6g/per 30g); prawns (14g/per 100g); tofu (12.6g/per 100g); feta cheese (16g/per 100g); flaxseed (6.6g/per 30g); chia seeds (5.5g/per 30g); pumpkin seeds (8.6g/per 30g) sunflower seeds (7g/per 30g); hemp seeds (11g/per 30g).

THE CARBSCALE

What is THE KETO DIET?

Keto is short for ketogenic, which as you can see from the CarbScale (below) is very low carb. Simply put, a ketogenic diet uses ketones as an alternative type of fuel, which are made in your liver from the breakdown of fats when glucose is in short supply.

Ketosis, using ketones as a fuel, is a natural state and one that is also used to make energy when you are fasting and not eating at all. This is a wonderful adaptation which allowed us to survive when our food supply was less predictable than it is today.

THE LOW-CARB PLATE

A practical way to follow a low-carb diet is to structure your plate around the different food groups:

For everyone:
* **Protein** – the hero of your plate
* **Non-starchy vegetables** (see page 28) – to add bulk, fibre (for good gut health) and vitamins
* **Added fats** – used in cooking or added for flavour, such as butter, olive oil, sauces

Then add extra carbs depending on your goals. Below is an example of how a meal can be tweaked depending on where you are on the CarbScale:

Chicken wrapped in bacon (see page 103), served with:
* **Keto** – celeriac, broccoli, tomato – 14g carbs
* **Strict** – celeriac, broccoli, tomato, plus an apple – 27g carbs
* **Moderate** – quinoa, broccoli, tomato – 45g carbs

One question you may have when thinking about moving to a low-carb diet is: how low should I go? This is a low-carb not a no-carb plan, as you will include slow-release carbohydrates and fibre from vegetables, fruit and pulses (beans and lentils). We use the CarbScale to help you identify the level that works best for you. Throughout this book we work on net carbs, which excludes the indigestible fibre in food: this helps to nourish your gut bacteria and doesn't impact your blood sugar levels.

As Dr Unwin mentions on page 5, low carb is described as under 130g net carbs a day. As this book is about weight loss, we are focusing on slightly tighter control to help you to better manage your appetite:

Moderate low carb = 75–100g net carbs per day. This enables a wide and varied diet and is a good starting point for eating low carb. It is also a good level for weight maintenance once you have achieved your weight-loss goals and are looking for a little more flexibility.

Strict low carb = under 50g net carbs per day. This gives you better glycaemic control, helping to keep your blood sugar levels stable and is a reasonable therapeutic target for weight loss, those with type 2 diabetes and if you have low energy or food cravings.

Keto = about 30g net carbs per day. A further reduction in carbs can be helpful if you are looking to lose weight quickly and are prepared to be stricter in order to meet your goals.

You can measure your carb intake, for instance using the nutritional analysis in these recipes or looking data up (see pages 204–205, or you could use a simple app – we like Carbs & Cals). However, it does not need to be complicated and you could instead just follow our Top 10 low-carb tips (see page 13).

The CARBSCALE (net carbs)

130g	120g	110g	100g	90g	80g	70g	60g	50g	40g	30g	20g	10g
Low carb (LC)			Moderate LC					Strict LC		Keto		

WHAT TO EAT
(and what not to eat)

1 **Reduce or eliminate starchy carbohydrates and sugars** from your diet, as both cause a rapid rise in blood sugar. These include breakfast cereals, bread, pasta, white potatoes, rice, couscous, crackers, oatcakes, rice cakes and also cakes, cookies, sweets, chocolate, fruit juice, fizzy drinks and cordials.

2 **Protein is a very important part of every meal**; it is used by your body for growth and repair. If you are vegetarian, then choose carefully to ensure you have an adequate protein intake from pulses, cheese, nuts, seeds and eggs. Omnivores also have the advantage of meat and fish, which are incredibly nutritious and good sources of vitamin B12, iron and essential fats.

3 **Here's the good news: you can include good fats**, which are essential for your metabolism and help you to feel fuller for longer. Oily fish such as salmon, mackerel, sardines and anchovies contain omega 3 which helps to reduce inflammation and keep your brain healthy. Olive oil can be used as a salad dressing and for very light frying. Butter, ghee, lard and coconut oil are all tasty saturated fats which are safe to heat in roasting and frying. Avoid margarines and vegetable oils, which oxidize when heated. Also avoid low-fat products, which tend to include sugars and sweeteners to improve flavour. Full-fat yogurt is a good choice.

4 **Focus on lots of vegetables with each meal.** Non-starchy and salad vegetables should be eaten generously so that you feel full at every meal (see page 28). You can still use gravy, curry and other sauces over your vegetables. Some popular replacements for starchy carbs include shredded cabbage cooked in butter (instead of tagliatelle), cauliflower rice and courgetti, but you can also just include more varieties of veg.

5 **Starchy veg are allowed with each meal but in a modest portion** – these tend to be veg that grow underground, such as carrots, parsnips, sweet potatoes and beetroot. Just have a small portion and only one of these per meal alongside plentiful non-starchy veg.

6 **Enjoy nuts and cheese in moderation**; they are nutritious and tasty but also highly calorific, so go slow if you want to lose weight and have them as part of a meal instead of snacking on them.

7 **When it comes to fruit, berries are a good choice** as they are naturally low in sugar. Other fruits depend on how you react to the sugars. Modest portions of fruit within a salad or alongside a main course can add flavour and interest. Try to avoid high-sugar tropical fruits, such as mango, pineapple and banana.

8 **Don't snack, unless choosing an ultralight meal (see page 36) instead of a meal.** Fasting between meals and overnight improves your sensitivity to insulin, which helps to keep your blood sugars steady. We are not designed to eat constantly: aim for three good meals and then stop. While fasting, your digestive system gets a rest, and your body can concentrate on other vital jobs such as keeping your immune system strong, balancing hormones and spring cleaning (detoxification!).

9 **Try to avoid diet and low-calorie drinks,** although these are better than their sugar-laden cousins. There are studies showing that sweeteners create hunger, leaving you vulnerable to making poor food choices. Instead enjoy fresh water, green, herbal and redbush teas and coffee.

10 **Plan some low-carb treats or desserts,** for instance at the weekends or for high days and holidays (see pages 182–203). You can flex this depending on your weight-loss goals so that you do not ever feel deprived. A good way to manage this is to alternate between phases of active weight loss and maintenance.

LOW-CARB SWAPS

Don't feel cheated – here are some delicious low-carb swaps you can make using this cookbook.

*high
carb*

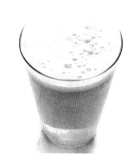 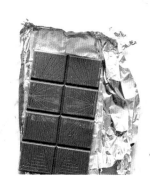

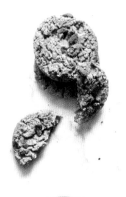 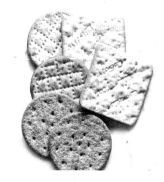 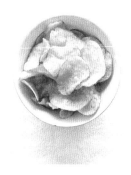

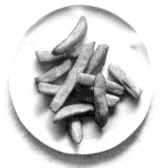 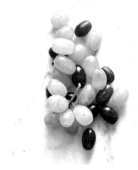 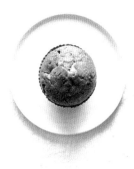

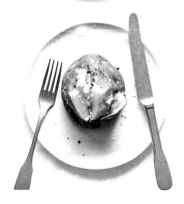 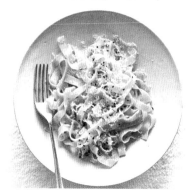 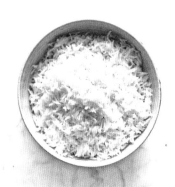

low carb

Red wine

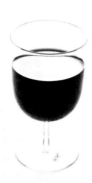

Dark chocolate (70%+ cocoa solids)

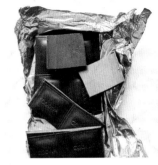

Roasted nuts

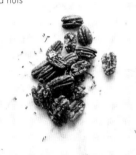

Super seed crackers
(page 73)

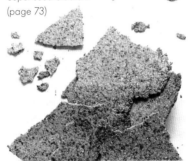

Cream cheese & peppers

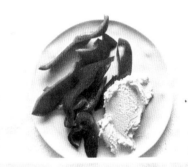

Root vegetable chips
(page 170)

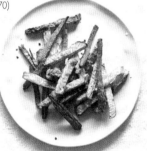

Low-sugar fruits

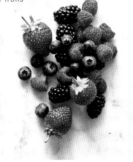

Cinnamon & cream cheese muffins
(page 48)

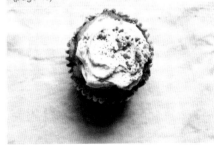

Roasted cauliflower

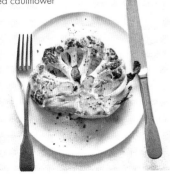

Cabbage pappardelle
(page 88)

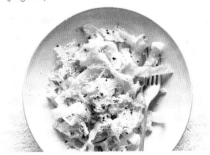

Cauliflower rice
(page 93)

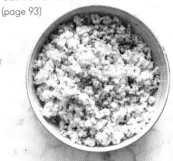

YOUR LOW-CARB FOOD PLANNER

Step 1 Choose your protein
Meat, fish, cheese, yogurt, eggs, nuts
& seeds, vegetarian e.g. soy

Step 2 Add non-starchy vegetables
Asparagus, aubergine, avocado, broccoli,
Brussels sprouts, cabbage, cauliflower, celery,
courgette, cucumber, fennel, garlic, green beans,
kale, leeks, lettuce, mangetout, mushrooms, okra,
olives, onions, peas, peppers, radishes, rocket,
spinach, string beans, tomatoes, watercress

Step 3 Add good fats and/or more carbs

	Add butter, oil or sauces	Add fruit	Add starchy veg	Include pulses, beans and lentils as protein
Keto (30g carbs)	✓	✗	✗	✗
Strict low carb (50g carbs)	✓	Up to one portion per day across these categories		
Moderate low carb (75–100g carbs)	✓	3–4 portions per day across these categories		

See the appendix on pages 204–205 to calculate the carbs in starchy vegetables, fruit and pulses

THE LOWDOWN ON ALCOHOL

While many of us enjoy an alcoholic drink, it is something
to savour in moderation if you are serious about losing
weight! Your best option is the odd glass of wine or spirits
with a low-calorie mixer. Beer and cider are unfortunately
very carby, hence the typical beer belly in regular
drinkers.

The first reason to go slow with alcohol is that it adds
extra calories, which will hinder your weight-loss efforts.
A large glass of wine (250ml/9fl oz) contains around
190 calories, which soon add up. More of a risk, though,
is that alcohol can lower your guard and ability to resist
the carby snacks which often go hand in hand with
socializing. Instead try to drink more water while you are
actively trying to lose weight, or herbal teas. You can add
lemon, ginger or cucumber for some subtle flavour, and
fizzy water is fine too.

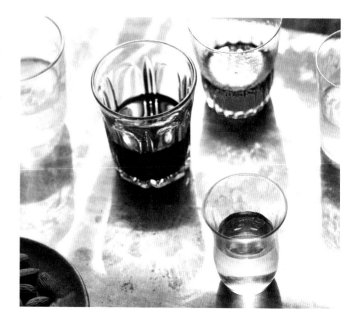

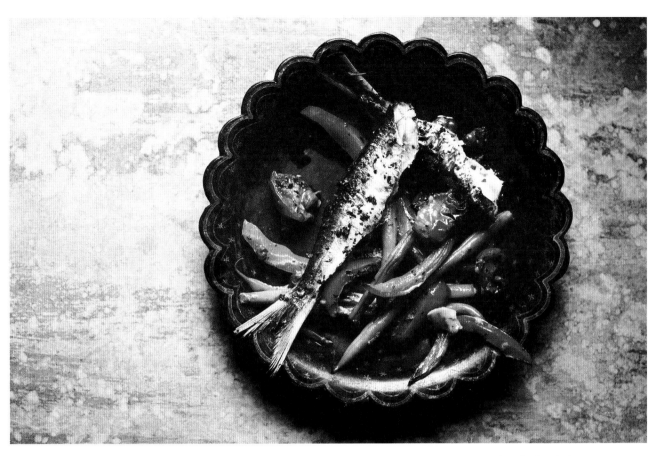

CARBS VS CALORIES

One of the big benefits of following a low-carb diet is freedom around eating, or at least a significant reduction in cravings. A study looking at the effect of two different diets on appetite over the course of a year backs this up. It found that measures of an appetite-stimulating hormone, peptide YY, was reduced in a low-carb diet versus a low-fat diet. This is great news because it makes it easier, and more enjoyable, to moderate your food intake when you are not hungry all the time.

The biggest impact you can make on reducing your calorie intake naturally is to eat low-carb meals which sustain you and stop snacking. Eat nothing between meals. Counting calories in foods can be very unhelpful

Low-fat, low-calorie foods tend to be very high in carbs, which don't sustain you.

when it encourages you to eat low-fat foods, because one way to drive down calories is to switch fats for carbs (because carbs contain fewer calories per gram than fat). But if you then end up eating foods that stimulate rather than satisfy appetite, you are likely to eat more throughout the day. This is borne out in the food diaries that I see, where three meals and multiple snacks is the norm for people struggling to lose weight.

To illustrate this point, consider how a filling low-carb breakfast of an omelette made with eggs, cheese and ham compares to a typical low-fat breakfast of porridge, toast, banana and orange juice. Both versions include a reasonable number of calories for a breakfast (471kcal vs 435kcal) – NHS health advice (UK) is to eat 2,000kcal a day (for a woman); 2,500kcal (for a man) – but the composition of the two meals is completely different. The low-calorie breakfast contains a whopping 70g carbs, which is roughly equivalent to 14 teaspoons of sugar! It contains 67 per cent less protein, and 63 per cent less fat than the low-carb breakfast. Fat and protein are satiating (they fill you up), whereas higher carbs promote hunger. If you ate the low-calorie breakfast, you would probably seek a mid-morning snack to "keep you going", whereas the low-carb option would keep you going far longer, and usually until at least lunchtime. The low-carb breakfast prioritizes protein and good fats over carbs, keeping insulin levels relatively low and hence enabling you to burn fat stores between meals. When you naturally don't feel hungry, weight loss is sustainable and enjoyable.

Omelette with ham (page 50)
2g carbs, 471 calories, 39g protein, 33g fat
Fast until lunch

vs

Porridge made with semi-skimmed milk,
with banana, one slice of toast with low-fat spread,
orange juice (150ml/5fl oz)
70g carbs, 435 calories, 13g protein, 12g fat
Plus a mid-morning snack as hunger levels kick in

We're not saying that calories don't count, it's just that food quality, and keeping carbs low, are more important. We have flagged the recipes as either ultralight, light or generous to help you avoid overeating low-carb foods. On the days that you have breakfast, you might like to choose both a light and a generous meal (no grazing in between!). When having brunch, opt for a generous meal, plus an ultralight meal in between if you feel you need it.

When you naturally don't feel hungry, weight loss is sustainable and enjoyable.

What about INTERMITTENT FASTING?

If you are currently used to grazing throughout the day, following advice to "eat little and often", you might feel concerned about the prospect of only eating meals and no snacks. This is known as intermittent fasting and is a very natural way to eat. Back in our caveman days, food supplies were very unpredictable, and times of feast or famine would have been the norm. There certainly wasn't a supermarket in walking distance!

Eating less often has lots of benefits for health, and the reason it works so well when you follow a low-carb diet is because you naturally feel less hungry. This really helps weight loss, simply because you have the opportunity to cut calories without compromising the quality of the meals you eat.

This plan recommends you start with three meals a day, aiming for about 5 hours in between each one. To accelerate your weight loss, you may find that you can even reduce this occasionally and enjoy just two meals a day, which extends the period that you are in a fasted state. Provided that you keep your carb intake low, then you should become more efficient at burning fat as a fuel. You can then start losing weight relatively effortlessly.

Before YOU BEGIN

If you are taking medications for diabetes or hypertension (high blood pressure), please discuss any change of diet with your doctor. They will then be able to monitor your progress and adjust your medications if required.

Make sure that you are adding salt generously to your meals. When you reduce your insulin levels through lowering your carbs you may feel a little light-headed. This is because insulin retains sodium in your blood and hence, while your kidneys adjust, you may need to compensate. You can add a little salt to water or bone broth but adding it to meals is also a great way to improve flavour.

GETTING STARTED
our top tips

1 Decide where you are on the CarbScale
Do you want to count your carbs or would you prefer to follow the broad principles? If you do want to count carbs, then download a useful app such as Carbs & Cals or MyFitnessPal (there are others). Or simply use the nutritional analysis in the recipes and appendix (see pages 204–205) to estimate your daily carb intake. If you are new to low carb, we suggest you start at under 100g per day (moderate) and go lower once you are feeling comfortable with your meal plan. You can restrict your carb intake further when you're ready, moving to strict low carb or keto (see the CarbScale, page 24).

2 Clear your cupboards…
…of carby food as best you can, or at least move them to a space where you can avoid them. This particularly applies to sweet things like cakes and cookies – tuck or chuck them away so that they won't tempt you. If your family are also keen to make a low-carb transition, then that is fantastic. If not, they can continue with their own choices without putting you under pressure.

3 Shop for low-carb ingredients
Stock up on meat, fish, eggs, dairy and lots of vegetables. Add storecupboard ingredients like nuts, seeds, olive oil, tahini and more – see page 39. Most ingredients are readily available in supermarkets, with the odd more speciality item available online.

4 Plan ahead
By thinking ahead, you allow yourself time to defrost something from the freezer or pop to the shops and pick up extra ingredients. Leaving things to the last minute could make things much harder and risks you falling back into old habits. Firstly, think about your current recipe repertoire and adapt it to low-carb principles (see page 25). Then start to introduce new recipes from this book and transition yourself into a delicious way of eating.

Each recipe you try and like can then easily be added to your collection. It is very easy to flick through cookbooks, enjoying the beautiful pictures but not necessarily trying out something new. Make a rule – every time you pick up this book, choose ONE recipe, decide when to have it, make a list of the ingredients you need and make it happen! We have included meal plans to inspire you (see pages 40–41).

5 Save time
Make extra portions to save on prep time, either by batch cooking (see page 38) or just simply using leftovers. For example, a salmon supper could be reused as a salmon salad the next day, with a tasty dressing (see page 180). Pre-cooking meat, such as a chicken, or even buying it ready-cooked, can save lots of prep time.

6 Flex for the family
Don't try to convert other family members if they are not keen. Instead flex your meals. If your family want roast potatoes with a Sunday roast, you can either add in some roast celeriac for you or substitute the potatoes with lots of veg. The same with pasta – you can add a Bolognese sauce to a pile of vegetables, buttered cabbage or courgetti. Delicious and super low carb!

7 Reward yourself (but not with food!)
We are used to using food as a reward, to celebrate and to make us feel better. Think about alternatives, especially as you start to hit your goals. Each time you lose a big number, treat yourself. This could be making some time for you, where you indulge in an activity that you enjoy. It might be reading a book, watching a film, going for a long walk, soaking in a hot bath, calling a friend. If you are saving money, for instance by buying less pre-packaged foods and wine, then build up a little treat fund – working towards a spa day, a massage, some new clothes or something else that is important to you.

Your HEALTH IMPROVEMENT tracker

Weight loss is not the only side effect of changing to low-carb eating. You might also like to track your health improvements by rating yourself now, and then after 4 weeks of enjoying a low-carb diet.

Rate yourself out of 10, where 1 is low and 10 is high:

	NOW	AFTER 4 WEEKS
Energy levels		
Concentration		
Sleep quality		
Mood		
Digestion		
Hormone balance		
Skin health		
Joint health		
Craving levels		

FLEXING YOUR PLAN
for sustained weight loss

Simply changing your diet to enjoy low-carb meals and restricting yourself to eating three meals per day is sufficient for most people to lose weight. However, sometimes you may hit a plateau, where your weight doesn't seem to budge.

The first thing is to realize that weight loss isn't strictly linear, and as long as your direction is downhill, then little bumps along the way are OK. For this reason, you might find it more helpful to weigh yourself once or twice a week rather than every day.

You need to be honest with yourself. Are you sneaking in extra calories without realizing it? These might be soft drinks, a glass of wine, the odd snack. We are so good at kidding ourselves that the only way to really know is to commit to recording everything that passes your lips! This is why we advocate keeping a food diary (see page 13). If the reason for the stall is around motivation, then we have great advice from Dr Jen Unwin on page 35 about how to successfully make long-term changes.

Evelyn's story
INTERMITTENT FASTING TO BANISH HUNGER

Evelyn balances home life with three grown-up sons and a full-time job as a marketing executive. The boys returning to university gave her a window to explore her diet and make changes to help her to lose weight.

"There was a time when I would be shocked if my weight hit 11 stone, but with a gentle creep over the years I hit 12 and then 12½ stone. Throughout the day I would feel more and more uncomfortable around my waistband. I felt dumpy and middle-aged – and knew that I needed to make changes.

I tried to keep off the sweet stuff and would always have a 'healthy' bowl of porridge for breakfast. But by mid-morning I was so hungry I could almost chew my own arm off, and toast was a quick grab. Lunch was a wrap and a salad. Later, when hunger set in again, I'd snack on something like a packet of crisps and diet cola, thinking that it was good as it has no calories. Biscuits woke up my appetite and I found it hard to stop at one.

I was pretty sceptical about low carb until I went to one of Jenny's presentations. I knew about insulin from working with diabetes drugs and realized that these focus on the disease rather than how to prevent it. I took one thing on board initially – have eggs for breakfast, which I took like medicine, every day. What happened was a revelation, for the first time I felt in control of my appetite and lost a little weight.

A year later I picked up with Jenny again. We were coming out of lockdown and I was concerned about the long-term effects on my health from being overweight. So, with friends for company, I started a 21-day reset. I quickly switched into two meals a day – a late morning brunch, like eggs and avocado with tomatoes or spinach, and an evening meal of protein and veg. Nothing in between. I felt great. Previously, I had such an energy slump after lunch I would have to put my head on my desk; that never happens now.

My weight loss was consistent, and I have levelled out at about 10½ stone. I won't even consider eating before noon – I'll stretch brunch out until 2pm if my diary allows. I have so much energy I've been able to join the gym."

Top tips FOR LASTING WEIGHT LOSS

1 **Be realistic** – a weight loss of just 1–2lb a week, consistently, will get you to your goal.

2 **Check your protein** – try to consume 60–80g (2¼–2¾oz) a day – more if you have a larger frame or are exercising hard. Check the appendix for nutrition data (see pages 204–205 or use an app like Carbs & Cals.

3 **Go keto** – try limiting your carbs to 30g per day. As your carbs reduce, you should feel less hungry as you are not spiking your blood sugars.

4 **Reflect on your activity** – how can you move more within your day? Counting your daily steps via your phone or using a smart watch can be very motivating.

5 **Consider a short, extended intermittent fast.** First up, try eating two meals a day twice a week – a brunch maybe with eggs and vegetables in the late morning followed by a dinner of protein and veg. Once you have mastered this, you could consider a 24-hour fast once a week: either from lunch or dinner on day 1 to lunch or dinner on day 2.

On an extended fast, drink plenty of water. You can also enjoy a couple of cups of tea or coffee with either a dash of milk, or 2 teaspoons of cream. On a 24-hour fast, I also like to have a large cup of bone broth with plenty of salt and pepper. Something to look forward to!

6 **Are your bowels moving?** If things have slowed down, then increase your intake of vegetables, including some raw, and try a slice of low-carb bread made with psyllium husks (see page 64). This adds mostly soluble fibre and bulk to help movement through your digestive system. You could also try some stewed apple as a pudding (try the Apple & cinnamon pie filling on pages 192–193 without the pastry).

Chris's story
THE LIFE-CHANGING POWER OF LOW CARB

Chris lives in New York and has transformed his health by using low-carb eating to keep his insulin levels stable, losing nearly 6 stone in the process.

"I had been overweight since college, even though I've always been active by lifting weights and running. Many times, I tried losing weight – 'eat less, move more' makes sense and sounds like it should work. But now I know why it doesn't.

For 16 years, I owned an art and picture-frame store downtown, which was next to a bakery, across from a pizzeria and with numerous coffee shops and delis within walking distance. I worked long hours and was on my feet the whole time. In the morning I would grab a coffee and a couple of rolls, later I'd pop to the bakery or local shop and often grab some pizza to perk me up into the evening. It is easy to eat a lot when you eat the wrong foods.

My rude awakening came five years ago when I was 51. I hadn't been on the scales for a long time and was shocked that I clocked in at nearly 20 stone, by far my heaviest. I felt out of shape and was winded when climbing stairs. It wasn't so easy to play basketball and soccer with my kids. Things had to change.

To start with I dropped colas and soft drinks; I was having up to ten cans a day. Quickly I lost 18lb, but then I plateaued. My big breakthrough came a couple of years later when a good friend recommended Gary Taubes's book Why We Get Fat. I was riveted. That weekend we were going to a Mexican restaurant to celebrate our daughter's sixteenth birthday and for the first time I changed my order – cutting out the carbs and enjoying chicken, beans and cheese instead.

I had no trouble sticking to a low-carb diet and in only two weeks it had a profound change in how I thought about food. The cravings were so much less, and I could manage them because I understood the process – how insulin makes you hungry and how carby food increases insulin levels. I also increased my protein considerably. I achieved my goal weight and have maintained it easily for the past three years. This way of eating has opened up a whole new world to me."

THE KEYS TO LASTING WEIGHT-LOSS

Dr Jen Unwin, Chartered Clinical and Health Psychologist

The keys to success with any long-term lifestyle change are mindset, managing habits and noticing what works for you. Even if the plan in this book were the best in the world (which I believe it is!), change doesn't happen by magic. You will need to make the changes and stick to them long enough to see the benefits. This can be challenging in today's crazy carb-filled world. Sugar is everywhere and seems central to any celebration these days. Choosing to live a little differently requires motivation and social skills. In my experience, there are people everywhere, even in our own families, who will try and nudge us back to eating sugar and junk food.

The good news is that the simple way to get rid of sugar cravings and stop overeating ultra-processed food for good is to give it up. The answer is simple but not always easy! Sugar acts quickly on the brain when we eat it, to give us a boost of the feel-good brain transmitters serotonin and dopamine. Just like alcohol, nicotine or other drugs, this is how sugar can become addictive over time. Unfortunately, our brains respond to a sugar high by knocking out a few receptors for these transmitters to keep in balance. The result is that we have more cravings and need more sugar to get the same "hit" the next time. It's a trap. Over time we feel worse for eating more sugar but need to get our fix by having another "dose". If you find yourself with cravings for sweet foods that are hard to resist, eating more and more carbohydrates and are always hungry, then it's time to think about quitting carbs or at least radically cutting them back. Just like a person who can't moderate their relationship with alcohol, some of us are much better off without sugar.

Research has shown that the foods people binge on are always highly processed. I can overeat anything sweet or salty that's high in refined carbohydrates but a

big steak with green beans will leave me totally satisfied. The reason for this is to do with how our ancestors survived lean times. We were driven to eat carbohydrate-rich foods when they were available in the autumn. These foods override fullness signals so we can gorge and get fat to live through winter. This mechanism is in the primitive part of our brains and is a powerful force! Our logical brains find it almost impossible to suppress this urge. Have you ever decided not to eat biscuits and then been unable to resist the urge to have one when you saw them later? I know I have.

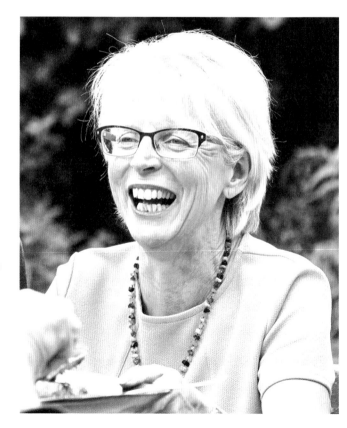

How to ESCAPE THE SUGAR TRAP

So how do we get out of this trap? There are three main steps. First, find your motivation. Second, set up your new habits and practise them until they are routine. Third, find new ways to boost those feel-good neurotransmitters in your brain so you aren't drawn back to sugar fixes. Let's look at each of these in turn.

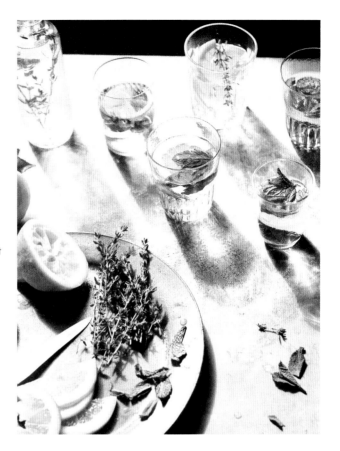

Motivation

What will keep you going when temptation strikes? What is it that you really, really want to achieve by changing the way you eat? Do you want more energy? To lose weight? To come off medications? Get fit? And what difference will it make to your life if you achieve these outcomes? How will life be better? What will you be able to do differently? This vision of a better future, the pot of gold at the end of the rainbow, is what will keep you going when times are challenging. Have a good long think about why changing the way you eat matters to you and maybe discuss it with family and friends to enlist their support.

Habit change

The next stage is changing your habits using preparation and planning. When will you start? What changes will you make? Be sure to clear all the junk and high-carb foods out of your house. It's much harder if they are close at hand. Fill your fridge and larder with nutrient-dense, low-carb foods. If other members of your household insist on keeping their "stash", then have a cupboard for yourself and a section of the fridge to make it clear what is your food. Prepare for the first couple of weeks carefully with shopping and meal planning so that you get in a routine right from the start. After the first couple of weeks, you will start to notice benefits, such as better sleep and more energy, not to mention weight loss, which will help to keep you motivated.

Happy hormones

When you are in a routine with meals and starting to feel in the swing of a low-carb life, that is the time to think about other changes that will make the habits you have begun more permanent. How might you get some happy hormones every day without resorting to sugar? Exercise is a fantastic way to boost dopamine and serotonin naturally. Exercising outdoors is especially beneficial. Walking is fine, or find another activity that you enjoy and can fit into your daily routine. Any form of relaxation or stress management will also help with weight loss and cravings. Yoga is a fantastic practice for brain health. Do you have time for a new hobby or to learn a new skill? I have taken up knitting in the evenings instead of eating!

It's normal and to be expected that you will struggle occasionally and may well fall off the wagon with your eating plan. The best way to deal with these times is to see them as lessons learned. Think about what triggered the problem. How might you deal with a similar situation differently next time? Quickly get back in the saddle and continue your journey!

THE RECIPES

Eating low-carb has become a way of life for Giancarlo and I for the past nine years; it has become a habit and I therefore have to remind myself what is important and different about the way we eat. Being low-carb doesn't alter the roast beef or the chicken tikka masala but it does alter the Yorkshire puddings and the pilao rice you have with them. With this in mind, I have concentrated on recipes that I consider useful: the sides that we eat instead of mashed potatoes, the what-to-have-instead-of-pasta recipes, how to make low-carb bread, and our essential carb swaps, the Carb Crushers as we call them (see pages 80–97).

All the recipes in this book are both sugar- and gluten-free. Since this book is about weight loss, nutritionist Jenny Phillips has encouraged me to make sure the recipes have adequate protein (see page 18). This contributes to her clients keeping to their weight-loss goals and not needing to snack between meals. Have a look at the photos on pages 20–23 to see which foods are the best sources of protein.

The recipes in the book span the CarbScale (see page 24) from keto up to moderate low-carb once your goal weight is achieved. I have given the nutritional analysis at the bottom of each recipe. As ingredients vary so much this is only a guide, but it will help you see the nutritional value of the meals in respect of carbs, protein and fats. You can use various software to calculate carbs (and there are discrepancies between them) or the Carbs & Cals app or book. Alternatively, I find it a good idea to look at what you are eating and imagine it as a pile of ingredients, or read the label – if it is made from low-carb ingredients, such as a few almonds, a vegetable, an egg, meat or fish with a little flavouring, then go ahead and eat it. If it was a pile of wheat flour or rice originally, poor-quality fat, sugar and various additives, then it will be high in carbs, so don't.

FLEXIBLE MEALTIMES

U ultralight

L light

Ⓖ generous

Every recipe has a symbol to say whether it is ultralight, light or generous to help you choose your meals appropriately. The chapters include breakfast but aren't specific to lunch and dinner, as most of us no longer eat in such a traditional way. Depending on what we've got on, we can now easily flex our mealtimes and frequency of eating. However, we don't snack between meals or graze our way through the day. Often Giancarlo and I skip breakfast or just have a coffee with cream and enjoy a generous brunch late morning, which keeps us powered for the day. If we have had a generous lunch out, we choose an ultralight meal in the evening as we aren't hungry for more. Feel free to mix and match these recipes to fit in with your schedule and commitments.

ULTRALIGHT MEALS

Hot buttered toast (page 51)
Sautéed greens with chilli & garlic (page 167)
Rainbow stir-fry (page 168)
Low-carb mash (page 173)
Baked "beans" (page 175)
Brussels sprout, bacon & leek hash (page 176)
Pilao cauli rice (page 93)
Mixed salad and classic vinaigrette (page 180)
Cooked chicken or turkey slices and a tomato
Giorgio's moutabal with sliced red pepper (page 148)
Boiled eggs with chopped celery
30g (1oz) cheese and a handful of olives
Bone broth (page 107)

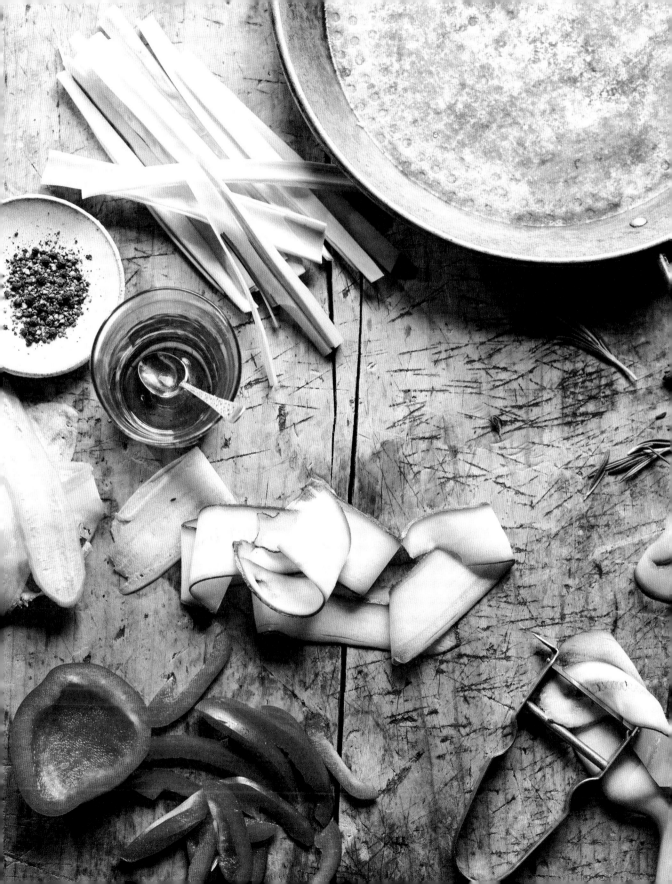

BATCH COOKING

Batch cooking means you can have your own healthy home-cooked meals in minutes. Safe food storage is all about limiting bacterial growth. Bacteria need moisture, air and warmth to grow, so by removing one or more of these elements you are making it harder for foods to spoil.

Cool hot food that is designed for storing quickly. It needs to be room temperature before putting in the fridge or it will heat up the rest of your food. Ideally get your leftovers in the fridge within 1½ hours. To speed up the cooling time, transfer hot food to a cold, shallow dish and stir frequently or put it into a bowl over another one full of iced water.

Reheating means cooking again, not just warming up. Always reheat food until it is steaming hot (70°C/158°F or above for at least 2 minutes) all the way through. If you use an oven, the heat is more evenly distributed than a microwave, where you might have some hot areas and others cold. However, microwaves are energy-efficient, so give your food a good stir halfway through reheating to distribute the temperature evenly.

Here are some ideal recipes for larger batches:
Chaffles (page 44)
Cinnamon & cream cheese muffins (page 48)
Coconut & ginger granola (page 57)
Chocolate orange pancakes (page 58)
Country-style loaf (page 64)
Brown bread baguettes (page 67)
White bread rolls (page 69)
Easy pizza (page 70)
Super seed crackers (page 73)
Coconut crêpes (page 79)
Bolognese ragù (page 85)
Cauli rice (page 93)
Ye olde pottage (page 100)
Mighty meatloaf (page 118)
Boeuf bourguignon (page 119)
Slow-cooked lamb curry (page 122)
Quick & spicy stir-fried lamb mince (page 125)
Fish & coconut curry (page 139)

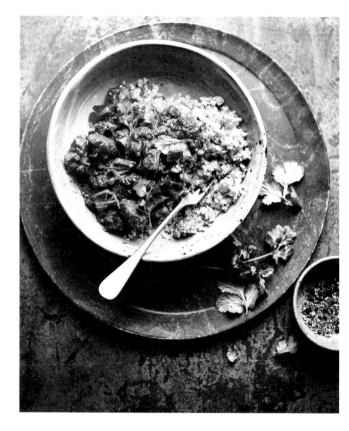

Aubergine parmigiana (page 147)
Saag-style kale & paneer (page 154)

TIME AND ENERGY-SAVING TIPS

Read the recipe all the way through before beginning – it saves time and resources in the end.

These recipes don't always start with preheating the oven. This is because, with an eye on energy efficiency, I now preheat my oven just minutes before I need it. Make a mental note of how long it takes for your oven to heat up – mine takes just 8 minutes to get to 220°C/200°C fan/425°F/gas mark 7, so there is no need for it to be on 30 minutes before I need it. You can also put food in the oven as it warms up.

Most households have a microwave and these only use a small amount of energy.

The LOW-CARB kitchen

You can always rustle up a quick dish without ever resorting to ready-meals
if you have these essential storecupboard ingredients to hand.

ALWAYS-IN-THE-FRIDGE FOODS

Greek yogurt

Double cream

Salted or unsalted butter ideally made from milk from
grass-fed cows – either is fine for any of the recipes

Parmesan or **Grana Padano**, **Cheddar** and **cream cheese**

Vegetables – cabbages, spring onions, lettuce, carrots,
peppers, aubergines, cucumber, celery, cauliflower

Lemons

Celery and the leaves from a bunch of celery. They can be
used anywhere instead of flat-leaf parsley and basil; try
them stirred into scrambled eggs or scattered over soups.

Harissa paste – seek out a good variety that you like,
made from chilli, salt and oil

Chipotle paste

Horseradish sauce

Nuts – pine nuts, walnuts, almonds, pecans and
macadamia are best stored in the freezer for instant
flavour and crunch

Flaxseed – golden gives a good colour to baking; keep
it in the fridge to stop it becoming rancid

Herbs – I always have coriander, parsley and thyme in
the fridge to liven up foods last minute

IN THE CUPBOARD

Baking powder – we look for a gluten-free version

Psyllium husk (coarse not powder) – available from
health food shops and online

Coconut flour – find it in larger supermarkets and health
food shops

Ground almonds

Erythritol

Inulin

Stevia

Vanilla extract – preferably without sugar but that can
be hard to find or expensive and I use a lot!

Frozen low-carb fruit

Canned beans, **lentils**, **chickpeas**

Canned tomatoes – a good Italian brand

Canned sardines, **mackerel**, **tuna** and **pilchards**

Dijon, **wholegrain** and **English mustard** – for an instant
low-carb kick

A range of vinegars – but actually just red wine or cider
vinegar would do and a medium-priced balsamic

Coconut oil, **ghee** (I make my own), **dripping** (saved fat
from roast meat)

Dried lentils, **chickpeas**, **beans**

Peanut butter

Tahini (sesame seed paste)

Tamari and **soy sauce**

Worcestershire sauce

Toasted sesame oil

Toasted sesame seeds (toast plenty and keep them in a
jar for instant flavour and crunch)

Spices – ground coriander, cumin and turmeric, curry
powder, chaat masala powder, chilli flakes, paprika,
smoked paprika, black onion (nigella) seeds, fennel seeds

BY THE HOB

Extra virgin olive oil – I keep two types, one standard
variety for cooking and one more expensive single-
estate oil for drizzling over cooked foods and salads

Black pepper from a good peppermill

Fine sea salt, preferably without an anti-caking agent,
as I believe you get a better distribution of flavour than
salt flakes, which are also expensive

Eggs – any size is good

Tomatoes – stored out of the fridge for the best flavour

Onions and garlic

For a more thorough list of low-carb ingredients,
sourcing and tips on cooking, see our website:
www.thegoodkitchentable.com

Meal plan – week 1

	BREAKFAST	LUNCH	DINNER	Total carbs
Mon	Granola, yogurt and berries, page 57 (15g carbs)	Mediterranean sardine bake, page 136 (10g carbs)	Ye olde pottage, page 100 (7g carbs) and 2 Sausage Rolls, page 72 (3g carbs)	35g
Tues	Chaffles, page 44 (3g) with 1 poached egg & avocado (1g)	Ye olde pottage, page 100 (7g carbs) and 2 Sausage rolls, page 72 (3g carbs)	Bolognese ragù on kale pezzi, page 85 (12g carbs) and 120g (4oz) strawberries (7g carbs)	35g
Weds	Granola, yogurt and berries, page 57 (15g carbs)	Green beanguine all'amatriciana, page 89 (17g carbs)	Slow-cooked lamb curry, page 122 with Pilao cauli rice, page 93 (14g carbs)	46g
Thurs	Chaffles, page 44 (3g carbs) with Baked "Beans", page 175 (4g carbs)	Leftover Slow-cooked lamb curry, page 122 with Pilao cauli rice, page 93 (14g carbs)	Easy pizza (freeze the extra bases), page 70 (6g carbs) with Spicy avocado salad, page 162 (8g carbs)	35g
Fri	Scrambled eggs & smoked salmon, page 52 (1g carbs)	Celery & Stilton soup, page 153, plus 1 slice of Country-style loaf, page 64 (4g carbs) plus 1 apple (14g carbs)	Leftover Bolognese ragù, page 85 (11g carbs) on Roast sprouts with cheese, page 86 (7g carbs)	37g
	BRUNCH			
Sat	Smoked salmon salad, page 128 (5g carbs)		**Dinner Party** Tuna, avocado & mango ceviche, page 132 (7g carbs), Aubergine parmigiana (with lamb mince), page 147 (21g carbs) with Sautéed Greens, page 167 (1g carbs) Mini pavlovas, page 196 (7g carbs) 2 glasses (175ml/6fl oz) of wine (2g carbs)	43g
Sun	Grilled portobello mushrooms with bacon, tomatoes & poached eggs, page 54 (12g carbs) Cinnamon & cream cheese muffin, page 48 (9g carbs)		Simple roast chicken with mushroom & cream sauce, page 104 (4g carbs) with Roast fennel & onions, page 165 (11g carbs) and celeriac mash, page 173 (8g carbs)	44g

Meal plan - week 2

	BREAKFAST	LUNCH	DINNER	Total carbs
Mon	Scrambled eggs, page 52, with Hot buttered toast, page 51 (2g carbs)	Lettuce cups with ham, chicken, tomatoes & mayo (using leftover roast chicken), page 108 (5g carbs)	Aubergine parmigiana (with lamb mince), page 147 (21g carbs) with 100g (3½oz) broccoli (2g carbs) 20g (¾oz) 85% dark chocolate (4g carbs)	34g
Tues (Fast day)	Coffee with cream (1g carbs)	Bone broth, page 107 (4g carbs)	Creamy cod & broccoli mornay, page 134 (7g carbs)	12g
Weds	The open omelette with ham, page 50 (2g carbs)	Cinnamon & cream cheese muffin, page 48 (9g carbs)	Swedish meatballs in cream sauce with berry jam, page 124 (6g carbs) with Brussels sprout, bacon & leek hash, page 176 (6g carbs)	23g
Thurs	Leftover Brussels sprout, bacon & leek hash, page 176, with 2 eggs (9g carbs)	Easy pizza (freeze the extra bases), page 70 (6g carbs) with Spicy avocado salad, page 162 (8g carbs)	2 high-meat-content sausages (1g carbs), 40g (1½oz) frozen peas (3g carbs) and swede mash, page 173 (3g carbs), plus 1 apple (14g carbs)	44g
Fri	Coconut & ginger granola, page 57, with yogurt and instant jam, page 47 (21g carbs)	Spiced aubergine with tomatoes & crispy onions on feta cream, page 144 (15g carbs)	Chicken souvlaki, page 112 (3g carbs) with Cucumber & tomato raita, page 181 (3g carbs) and Spicy avocado salad, page 162 (8g carbs) 2 glasses (175ml/6fl oz) of wine (2g carbs)	52g
	BRUNCH			
Sat	Tamari mushroom bowl with 100g (3½oz) cooked chicken, page 149 (7g carbs)		Fish & coconut curry, page 139 (12g carbs) with Cauli rice, page 93 (6g carbs) Stefano's squidgy chocolate mousse cake, page 191 (4g carbs)	29g
Sun	Chocolate orange pancakes with yogurt & raspberries, page 58 (16g carbs)	Slow-cooked pulled pork, page 116 (5g carbs) with Super slaw with mustard dressing, page 166 (10g carbs) and 1 Strawberry & vanilla verrine, page 200 (7g carbs)	Super seed crackers, page 73 (3g carbs) with 75g (2¾oz) cheese (0g carbs), plus 1 apple (14g carbs)	55g

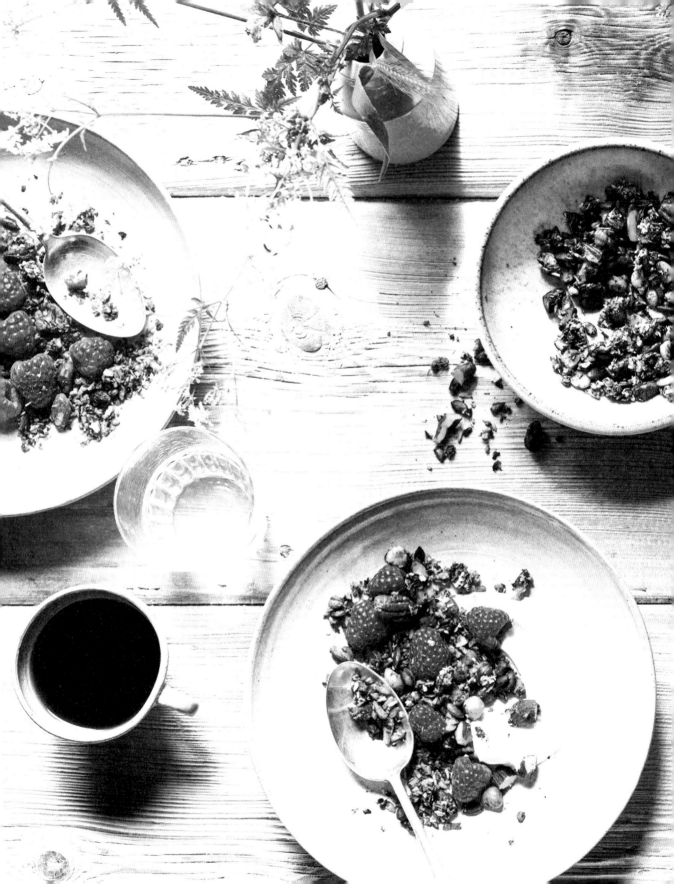

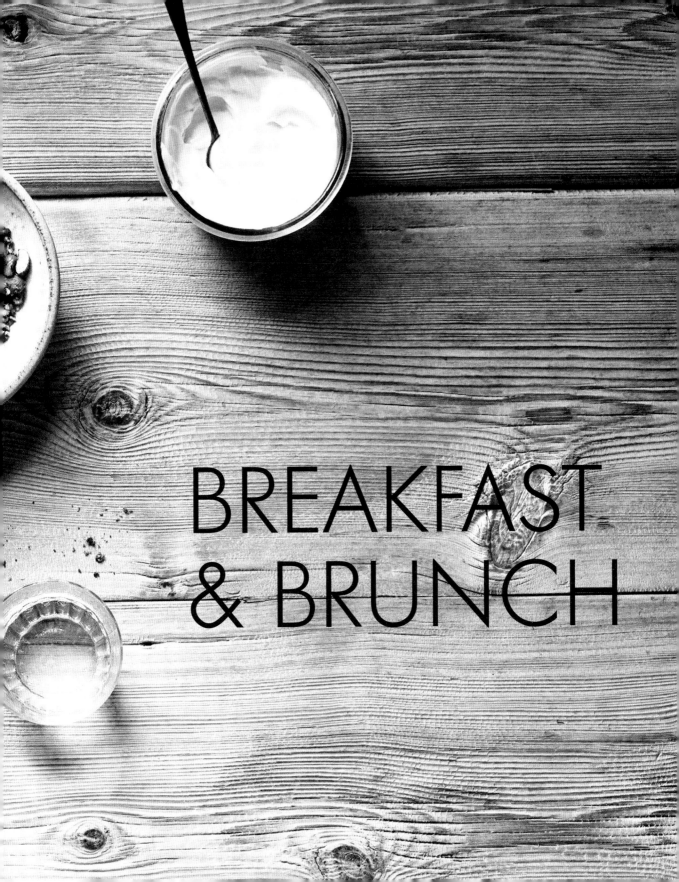

BREAKFAST & BRUNCH

CHAFFLES

L

SERVES 2/MAKES 1 LARGE OR
2 SMALLER CHAFFLES

2 eggs
40g (1½oz) mature Cheddar cheese,
    coarsely grated
40g (1½oz) ground almonds
½ teaspoon baking powder

Toppings
Baked "beans" (page 175)
whipped cream cheese and chives
bacon slices
avocado slices and lime
finely sliced green chillies

Per chaffle
3.4g net carbs, 2g fibre,
14.9g protein, 22.6g fat, 285kcal

Per chaffle with 10g (¼oz) butter
3.4g net carbs, 2g fibre,
14.9g protein, 26.7g fat, 320kcal

Per chaffle with ½ avocado and
2 tablespoons of cream cheese
5.9g net carbs, 6.3g fibre,
17.5g protein, 35g fat, 427kcal

These cheesy waffles known as "chaffles" have become fashionable in the low-carb community as quick meal bases. They take minutes to make and have so many possible toppings I could write a whole book about them! If you don't have a waffle maker, the mixture makes American-style pancakes in a non-stick frying pan with a little oil. If you have a sandwich maker, the mixture works in those too. To alter the flavour, try adding a teaspoon of chopped herbs, such as chives or thyme, to the mixture.

Chaffles make a good breakfast freshly made or warmed in the toaster directly from the fridge or freezer. Spread with a little butter and Marmite, two chaffles give you enough protein to last you through to lunch. Alternatively, try one topped with the Baked "beans" from page 175 and a poached egg.

Heat your waffle maker. Mix the eggs, grated cheese, ground almonds and baking powder together thoroughly and pour into the waffle maker. Depending on your waffle maker, the mixture makes 1 large or 2 smaller chaffles. Close the lid and wait for 3–6 minutes, depending on the efficiency of the waffle maker. When it stops steaming, your chaffle is done, so pay close attention. Lift the lid carefully and check the chaffles are golden brown, firm to the touch and therefore ready.

Top with your chosen toppings and enjoy.

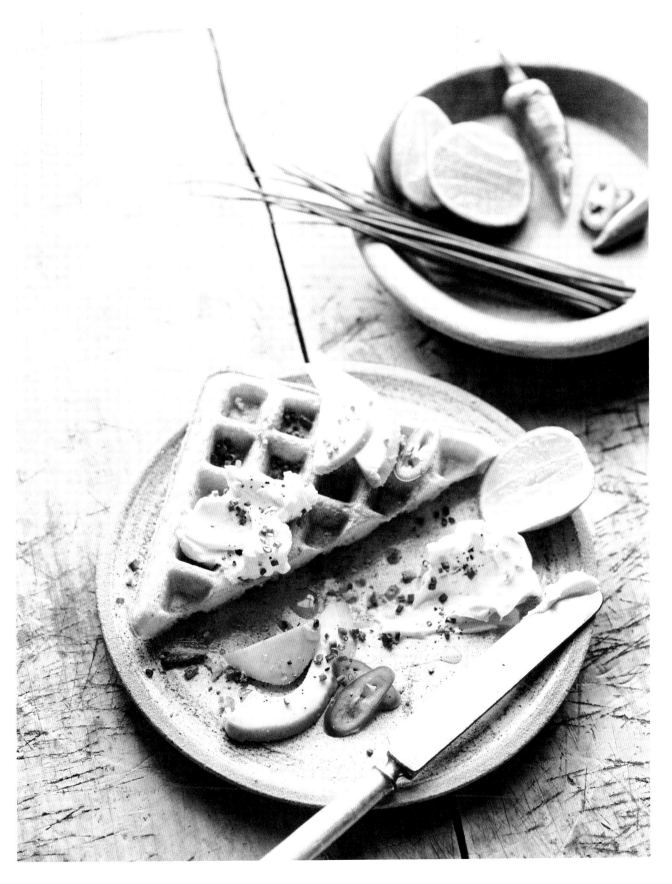

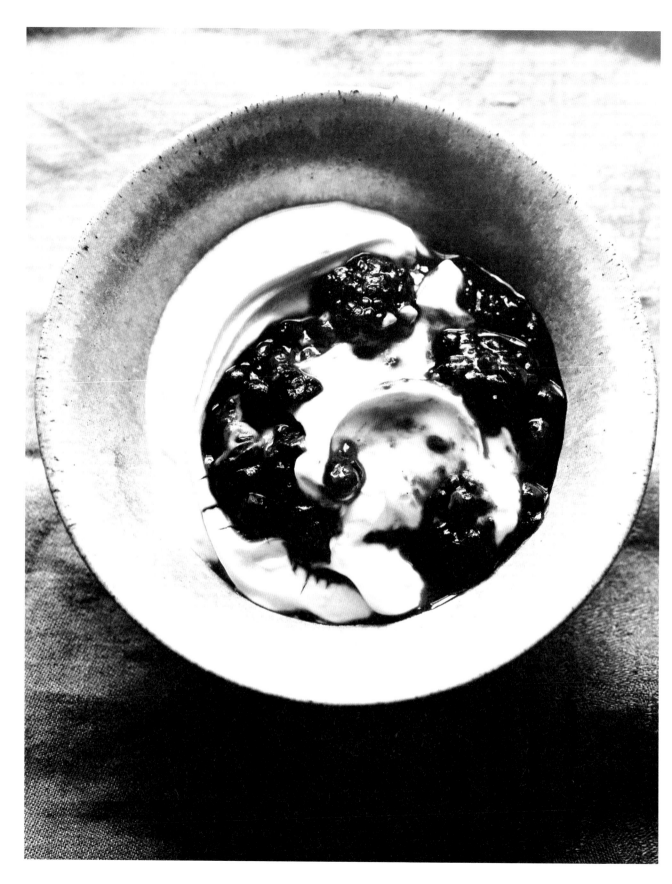

YOGURT SWIRL WITH INSTANT JAM

L

SERVES 4/ MAKES 200G
(7OZ) COMPOTE

200g (7oz) mixed frozen berries,
    such as raspberries, strawberries,
    blueberries, blackberries or currants

1 star anise (optional)

2 strips of orange peel (optional)

2 tablespoons orange juice

1 teaspoon vanilla extract, to taste

3 tablespoons powdered erythritol
    or 1 tablespoon honey

To serve

600g (1lb 5oz) 10% fat Greek yogurt

Per serving
of Instant jam with honey
9.1g net carbs, 1.8g fibre,
0.4g protein, 0.2g fat, 48kcal

of Instant jam with erythritol
4.7g net carbs, 1.8g fibre,
0.4g protein, 0.2g fat, 32kcal

of 150g (5½oz) yogurt
6.8g net carbs, 0g fibre,
9g protein, 15g fat, 198kcal

Thick Greek yogurt and berries makes a super-simple breakfast, which is also filling, low in carbs and quick. To make it more substantial, add a handful of Coconut & ginger granola from page 57 or have a slice of Hot buttered toast from page 51 afterwards.

Commercial brands of sweetened yogurt can contain up to 20g (¾oz) carbs per 150g (5oz) serving, so even if you end up adding honey to the jam, it will still contain a lot less sugar than a ready-made version. When the jam is cool, transfer it to a jar and keep it in the fridge for up to 4 days. Although I like erythritol for flavour, it can cause problems as it can re-crystallize in recipes where there is a lot of liquid. To combat this, grind it to a powder in a small blender before using.

To make this in an instant, put all the ingredients in a microwave-proof bowl and heat on full power for about 3 minutes or until the berries are soft and begin to collapse.

Alternatively, put all the ingredients into a saucepan with 2 tablespoons of water and bring to the boil over a medium–high heat, stirring frequently. When the berries are soft, they are done. This should take about 5–7 minutes.

Any stubborn, larger berries, such as blackberries, can be mashed with a potato masher. Tip them into a bowl and leave to cool to room temperature. Serve swirled through the yogurt.

SIMPLE VERSION

L

150g (5½oz) 10% fat
    Greek yogurt

50g (1¾oz) fresh berries,
    such as raspberries
    or strawberries

1 teaspoon vanilla extract

Mash the berries into the Greek yogurt. It might sound silly, but the flavour really comes out when you mash the berries, and to give a little sweetness, add a teaspoon of vanilla extract. Serve straight away or chill in the fridge until you are ready to eat.

Per serving
15.9g net carbs, 1.8g fibre, 9.4g protein, 15.2g fat, 246kcal

CINNAMON & CREAM CHEESE MUFFINS

L
MAKES 6

3 eggs

150g (5½oz) ground almonds

1 (125g/4½oz) apple,
 coarsely grated

1½ teaspoons baking powder

1 tablespoon vanilla extract

For the cinnamon butter

45g (1½oz) butter, plus extra
 for greasing (optional)

3 teaspoons ground cinnamon

1 tablespoon honey or 2 tablespoons
 erythritol

For the cream cheese frosting

90g (3¼oz) cream cheese

2 teaspoons vanilla extract

Per muffin with honey
9.1g net carbs, 3.2g fibre,
8.8g protein, 27g fat, 322kcal

Per muffin with erythritol
7g net carbs, 3.2g fibre,
8.8g protein, 27g fat, 314kcal

When I worked as an au pair in Long Island, New York, cinnamon rolls were my downfall. I came back two stone heavier and haven't touched one since. However, I can now enjoy them once more with this low-carb version. I think these are much nicer than their sickly-sweet forebears, which can weigh in at 125g (4½oz) carbs and 880kcal each compared to mine at under 10g (¼oz) and 322kcal! These are great to freeze; defrost in the microwave and top with the cream cheese frosting before serving.

Preheat the oven to 220°C/200°C fan/425°F/gas mark 7. Grease 6 muffin moulds or use a silicone muffin mould or line a muffin tin with paper cases.

Mix the eggs, ground almonds, grated apple, baking powder and vanilla together thoroughly in a bowl. Use a spatula to transfer the mixture to the muffin moulds and smooth down the tops.

Bake the muffins for 20 minutes or until firm to the touch.

Meanwhile, make the cinnamon butter by mixing all the ingredients together and set aside. Do the same with the frosting.

Once cooked, use a thick skewer to make 3 holes in the top of each muffin. I circle the skewer around a little to enlarge the holes. Pour the warm cinnamon butter over the tops of the muffins so that each will be marbled with it. Set aside to cool.

Use a dinner knife or small spatula to spread the frosting over the muffins and serve straight away or keep the muffins in a container in the fridge for up to 4 days.

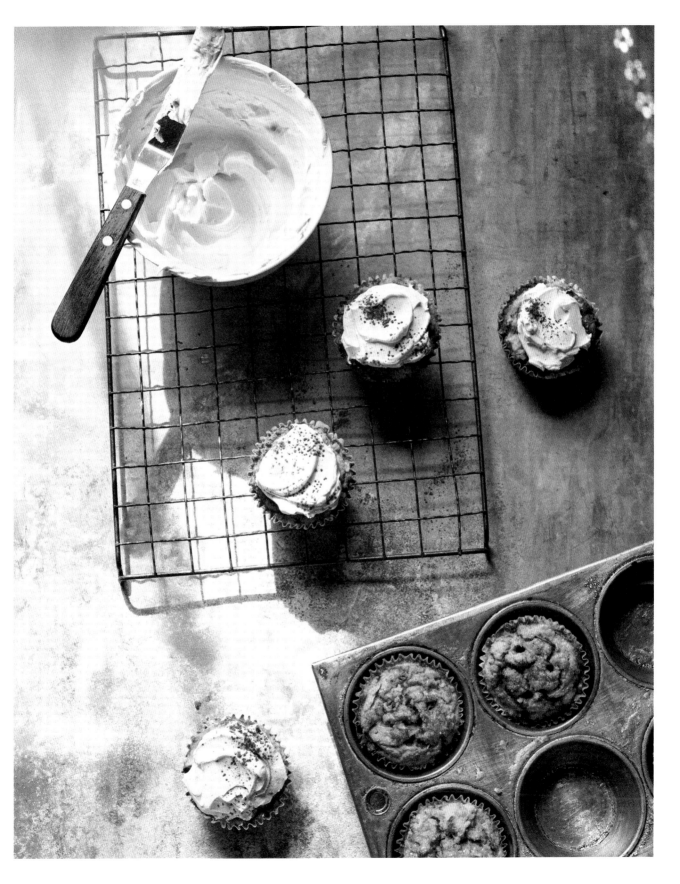

THE OPEN OMELETTE

L "keep it simple"

G with ham

SERVES 1

2 eggs

a knob of butter

a small handful of fresh herbs,
    such as dill, flat-leaf parsley
    or coriander, roughly chopped

100g (3½oz) cooked ham, bacon,
    chicken, roughly chopped
    (optional)

20g (¾oz) Cheddar cheese, grated

a few drops of hot sauce or a
    pinch of chilli flakes (optional)

salt and freshly ground black pepper

___

Per omelette
"keep it simple"
2g net carbs, 0.4g fibre,
16.1g protein, 24.2g fat, 293kcal

with ham
2g net carbs, 0.4g fibre,
38.7g protein, 33.2g fat, 471kcal

Rather than the traditional folded-over version, I have come to love these simple open omelettes. They are easy to make in minutes and great for using up leftovers from the fridge. I have included 75g (2¾oz) cooked meat to make sure the protein is adequate so that you are full until lunchtime, but you could use cooked or smoked salmon or tuna instead.

The herbs are interchangeable too, but I love to add them for colour and to get more plant diversity into my diet. If I have roasted vegetables in the fridge, then I add those too and top with cheese. For further omelette inspiration, look at *The Reverse Your Diabetes Cookbook* and *The 30 Minute Diabetes Cookbook*.

Make sure you have a warm plate ready and everything you need to hand to work quickly.

Crack the eggs into a bowl, add plenty of black pepper and a pinch of salt and whisk with a fork.

Melt the butter in a non-stick frying pan (with a lid) over a medium heat. Swirl it around to coat the base of the pan. Increase the heat to medium–high and add the eggs. Use a spatula to move the eggs around for about a minute, criss-crossing the pan to get the runny eggs to the bottom. Then leave it to set for about a minute, making sure there are no holes in the omelette. When the outer edges become opaque, run the spatula around the rim of the pan to loosen it. Shake the pan to make sure the omelette can slide.

Scatter the herbs, meat, if using, and cheese over the omelette and cover the pan with the lid. Cook for 2 minutes or until the eggs are cooked to your liking. Serve straight away with some hot sauce or a scattering of chilli flakes, if you wish.

HOT BUTTERED TOAST

U

MAKES 4 x APPROX. 6CM
(2½IN) CIRCLES OR 2
RECTANGULAR SLICES

1 tablespoon butter, softened, plus
    extra for greasing (optional)

3 tablespoons ground almonds

1 medium or large egg

a pinch of salt

¼ teaspoon baking powder

Per serving
(2 circles or 1 rectangle of bread)
1.3g net carbs, 1.1g fibre,
5g protein, 13.4g fat, 145kcal

Per serving
(2 circles or 1 rectangle of bread
buttered)
1.3g net carbs, 1.1g fibre,
5g protein, 16.2g fat, 171kcal

There are many ways to cook this bread depending on what you want to do with it afterwards and how you are going to eat it. If I want to make a sandwich, I use a small rectangular container, such as one used for cream cheese, to cook the bread in so that I can cut it into slices.

This bread is very low in carbs and calories, so enjoy it with scrambled eggs, buttered with Marmite or slathered with cream cheese and topped with smoked salmon to make sure it is filling so you aren't snacking between meals.

Mix all the ingredients together thoroughly in a small bowl, then transfer to a microwavable standard-sized mug or rectangular container measuring about 12 x 9cm (4½ x 3½in). (There is no need to grease it.)

Make sure the mixture is pushed down to the bottom of your chosen container to avoid air pockets. Microwave it on full power (for a 900W microwave) for 1 minute 20 seconds, or until cooked through and firm to the touch. Turn the bread out and leave to cool for a couple of minutes.

Use a serrated knife to cut the bread horizontally into 2 or 4 slices and eat as it is or toast it until golden brown and crispy.

If you don't have a microwave, preheat the oven to 220°C/200°C fan/ 425°F/gas mark 7. Lightly grease 2 ramekins or a small rectangular meatloaf tin with butter and put a circle of baking parchment on the bottom of each one. Divide the mixture between the 2 ramekins or pour it all into the tin. Bake for 10 minutes until golden brown and firm to the touch. Remove from the oven and leave to cool for 5 minutes before turning out. Cut the bread into slices and eat as it is or lightly toast in a toaster.

The bread will keep in a container or sealed bag for up to 4 days in the fridge.

SCRAMBLED EGGS & SMOKED SALMON

L

SERVES 2

2 eggs

1 tablespoon chopped flat-leaf parsley, coriander or celery leaves

10g (¼oz) butter, extra virgin olive oil or ghee

100g (3½oz) smoked salmon

a good pinch of salt and plenty of black pepper

lemon wedges, to serve

Per serving
1.1g net carbs, 0.1g fibre,
11.2g protein, 17.4g fat, 208kcal

with 50g (1¾oz) smoked salmon
1.1g net carbs, 0.1g fibre,
20.3g protein, 19.6g fat, 267kcal

Who doesn't love creamy scrambled eggs? At just over 1g of carbs, it's the perfect quick breakfast to set you up for the day. We like to mix herbs into it and then serve it in bowls with the simple addition of tomatoes and a dash of olive oil. The smoked salmon makes it more substantial, or you can swap this for bacon and mushrooms. It makes a great meal at any time of day and is lovely with the Hot buttered toast on page 51.

Use a fork to beat the eggs with the herbs and seasoning in a small bowl.

Melt the butter in a large non-stick frying pan over a medium heat until it starts to foam. Pour in the egg mixture and stir continuously with a wooden spoon as it begins to set. Move the runny eggs and solid areas together until the eggs are cooked to your liking. Remove from the heat and serve straight away with the smoked salmon and a wedge of lemon alongside.

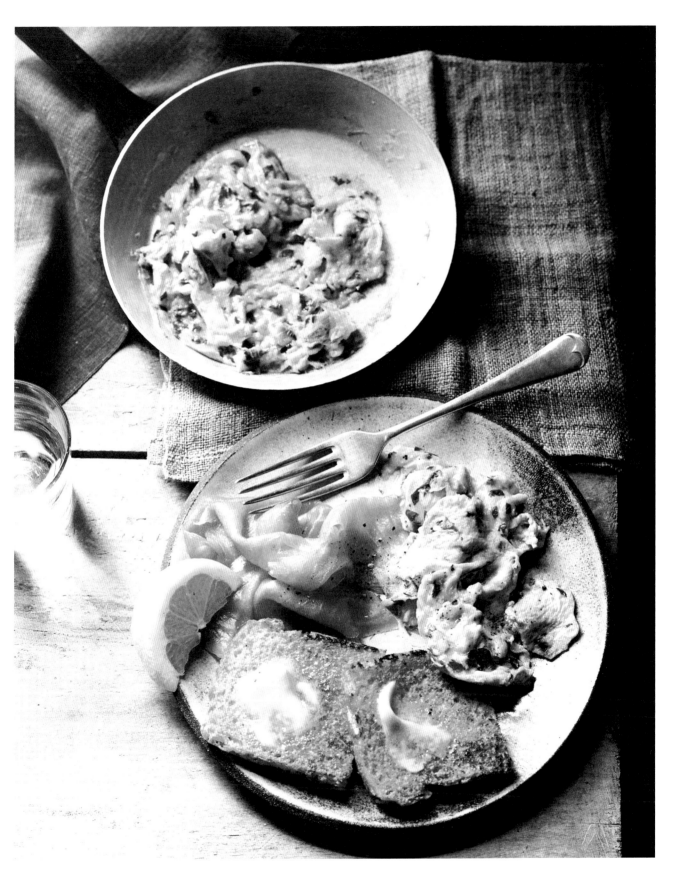

GRILLED PORTOBELLO MUSHROOMS WITH BACON, TOMATO & POACHED EGGS

SERVES 2

4 medium portobello mushrooms (approx. 250g/9oz), brushed clean

3 tablespoons extra virgin olive oil, plus a drizzle to serve

6 rashers of smoked streaky bacon

2 tomatoes or 6 cherry tomatoes, halved

4 eggs

salt and freshly ground black pepper

Per serving
12.2g net carbs, 6g fibre,
24.6g protein, 32.5g fat, 452kcal

Portobello mushrooms make the perfect low-carb base when wheat-based toast is off the menu. They take about 10 minutes to prepare under the grill and are so versatile. Either go for two giant portobello or four medium ones. Use grilled halloumi instead of bacon for a vegetarian option.

Preheat the grill to high. Bring a medium saucepan of water to the boil.

Cut away and discard the mushroom stalks. Lay the mushrooms gill-side up on a baking tray, brush with the oil and season with salt and pepper. Lay the bacon rashers and tomatoes next to the mushrooms. Grill, close to the heat source, for 6 minutes, or until the mushrooms are tender and darker around the edges. Turn the bacon when cooked on one side, then remove when cooked to your liking and set aside.

To poach the eggs, reduce the heat under the saucepan and let the water simmer gently. Crack one of the eggs into a teacup and partially submerge the cup in the water. Let the egg slide out into the water, disturbing it as little as possible. Do the same with the remaining eggs. Allow 3–5 minutes depending on how you like your eggs and lift them out one at a time with a slotted spoon. Set aside on a warm plate until you are ready to serve.

Use tongs to turn the mushrooms over so the bottoms are facing upwards and grill for a further 3 minutes, then transfer to warm plates. When the tomatoes are also done, remove and set aside with the bacon.

Arrange the mushrooms, bacon and tomatoes on 2 plates, then top each one with an egg. Finish with a scattering of pepper and a pinch of salt on each egg. Serve straight away.

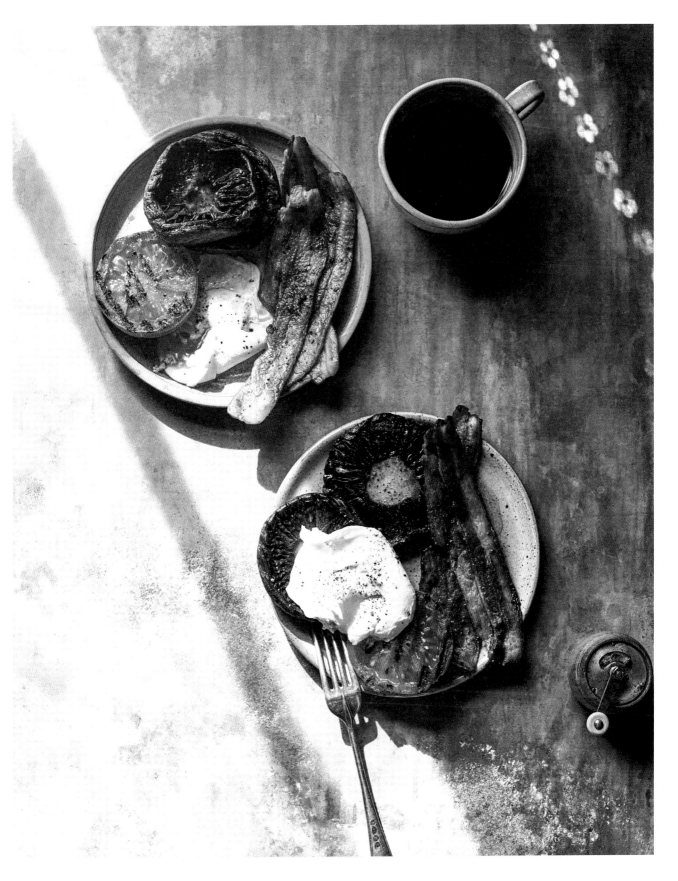

ASPARAGUS & POACHED EGGS WITH LEMON BUTTER

L

SERVES 2

200g (7oz) asparagus spears

1 tablespoon lemon juice (approx. ½ small lemon)

20g (¾oz) butter

4 eggs

10g (¼oz) Parmesan shavings

salt and freshly ground black pepper

Per serving
4.3g net carbs, 2g fibre,
15g protein, 19.1g fat, 252kcal

We love this any time of day when asparagus is in season. It also makes a good first course, in which case I would only serve one egg per person.

Snap the woody stems off the asparagus. Steam or boil the asparagus for 5–8 minutes until tender; the timing will depend on the width of the stalks. Drain and set aside on 2 warm plates or in shallow bowls.

Meanwhile, heat the lemon juice and butter together for a few minutes in a small pan or in a bowl in the microwave. Whisk together with a fork and season to taste.

Poach the eggs; I find this easiest to do in a large frying pan. Boil enough water in the pan so that the eggs have space to cook. When the water is simmering gently, crack one of the eggs into a teacup and partially submerge the cup in the water. Let the egg slide out into the water, disturbing it as little as possible. Do the same with the remaining eggs. This method allows you to poach several eggs at once depending on the size of your pan. Cook for 3–5 minutes, depending on how you like your eggs. Remove them with a slotted spoon, allowing any water to fall away.

Lay the eggs over the asparagus, pour over the lemon butter and finish with a little salt, a twist of black pepper and the Parmesan shavings.

COCONUT & GINGER GRANOLA

L

SERVES 6

15g (½oz) coconut oil or
    unsalted butter

1 egg white, lightly beaten

2 heaped tablespoons erythritol or
    1 tablespoon honey

75g (2¾oz) mixed nuts, such as
    pecans, walnuts, almonds,
    hazelnuts or macadamia,
    roughly chopped

50g (1¾oz) mixed seeds, such as
    pumpkin, sunflower or sesame

25g (1oz) fresh ginger, peeled and
    finely grated (optional)

15g (½oz) desiccated coconut

1 teaspoon vanilla extract

2 teaspoons ground cinnamon

Greek yogurt and low-carb berries,
    such as raspberries, blackberries
    or blueberries, to serve

Per serving
(approx. 25g/1oz) with erythritol
4.6g net carbs, 2g fibre,
4.4g protein, 16.3g fat, 173kcal

(approx. 25g/1oz) with honey
4.5g net carbs, 2g fibre,
4.4g protein, 16.3g fat, 180kcal

I used to be an oats-and-banana-every-morning kind of girl, but I was always hungry again by mid-morning. I now realize my "healthy breakfast" was full of sugar from the fruit, oats, honey, low-fat yogurt and skimmed milk. Since discovering a low-carb lifestyle, I don't crave breakfast until mid-morning or sometimes not at all, and when I do have it, this is one of my favourites. We also eat this in small quantities as a pudding.

Usually granola contains sugary dried fruits, honey or added sugar, but my granola relies on the natural sweetness of coconut and vanilla and the comforting warmth of ginger. I have used erythritol for just a hint of sweetness, but if you prefer to keep it natural, add minimal honey instead. If you don't have time for breakfast at home, take a serving of this in a container and eat it with coffee at work.

Preheat the oven to 200°C/180°C fan/400°F/gas mark 6 and line a baking tray with a silicone baking mat or baking parchment.

Melt the coconut oil in a small bowl in the microwave or in a small saucepan. Then mix it into the remaining ingredients in a large bowl and stir thoroughly. Taste the mixture and adjust with vanilla, sweetener or ginger as necessary.

Spread the mixture out over the prepared baking tray and cook for 8–10 minutes, or until the egg white has set and the nuts are lightly browned. Keep an eye on it, as coconut burns quickly, and give the tray a shake halfway through cooking to move the granola around and stop the outsides burning.

Remove the granola from the oven and leave to cool. It can be stored in a jar out of the fridge for up to 3 days or for up to a week in the fridge. To serve, scatter over yogurt with berries, or enjoy with whipped cream and cooked apple for dessert.

CHOCOLATE ORANGE PANCAKES WITH YOGURT & RASPBERRIES

L

MAKES 6 PANCAKES/SERVES 3

2 teaspoons coconut oil,
   ghee or butter

2 teaspoons vanilla extract (optional)

300g (10½oz) Greek yogurt or
   whipped cream (optional)

300g (10½oz) raspberries

For the pancakes

3 eggs

1 teaspoon vanilla extract

1 teaspoon baking powder

3 tablespoons coconut flour

2 tablespoons cocoa powder

2 teaspoons honey or
   30g (1oz) erythritol

30g (1oz) dark chocolate, 85%
   cocoa solids, roughly chopped

1 teaspoon finely grated orange zest
   (optional)

3 tablespoons water

Per pancake with honey
5.3g net carbs, 1.9g fibre,
4.2g protein, 6.9g fat, 101kcal

with erythritol
3.3g net carbs, 1.9g fibre,
4.2g protein, 6.9g fat, 94kcal

yogurt & berries
4.6g net carbs, 3.3g fibre,
4.6g protein, 1.3g fat, 59kcal

These pancakes were our son Flavio's idea. He works as a chef and heads off to the kitchen in the early hours of the morning. He asked me to create a chocolate pancake that he could grab from the fridge and take in a bag to work. I find one is enough for a light breakfast, but you can eat two if you're hungry.

These pancakes have the advantage of being nut-free (if you can eat coconut), gluten-free and lactose-free depending on your choice of chocolate. They are great as they are, or with berries, homemade vanilla yogurt, the Instant jam on page 47 or whipped cream. You can decide if you want to use an artificial sugar like erythritol to reduce the carbs or keep it natural with honey. They keep well too, so do make a batch and store them in the fridge for up to 3 days or the freezer for up to 3 months.

Whisk all the pancake ingredients together in a mixing bowl until thoroughly combined. The mixture should be a thick, dropping consistency; if it isn't, then add another tablespoon of water and stir through.

Heat a large non-stick frying pan over a low–medium heat and add 1 teaspoon of the coconut oil. When melted, swirl the oil around the pan to coat it. Drop 2 heaped tablespoons of the batter into the pan to make each pancake. Make sure they don't touch as they spread out; do this in batches if necessary, using the remaining teaspoon of coconut oil to grease the pan. Use a fish slice or spatula to gently turn the pancakes when they are set and firm around the edges. Don't worry if they darken underneath, they still taste delicious. They take 3–4 minutes on the first side and only 1–2 minutes on the second.

Remove the pancakes from the pan when cooked and serve straight away or keep warm while you make the others. Stir the vanilla into the yogurt, if using, and serve with the berries.

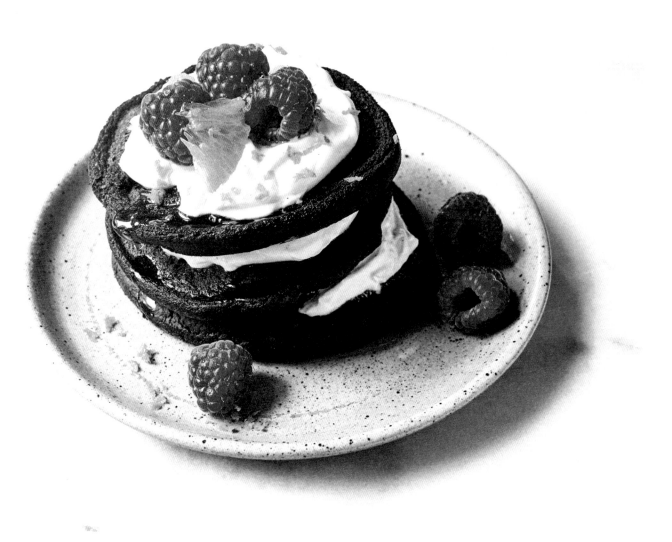

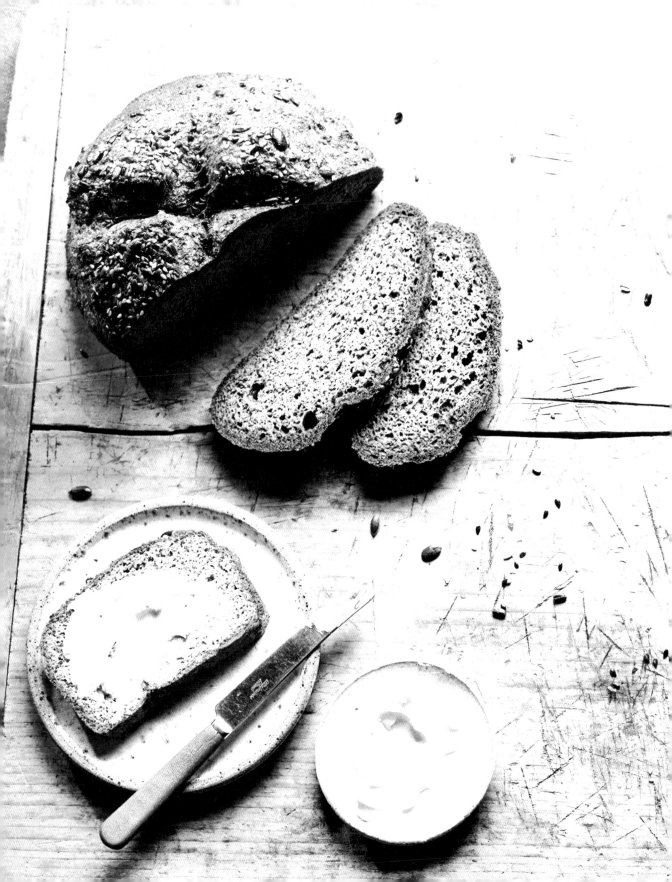

BAKING

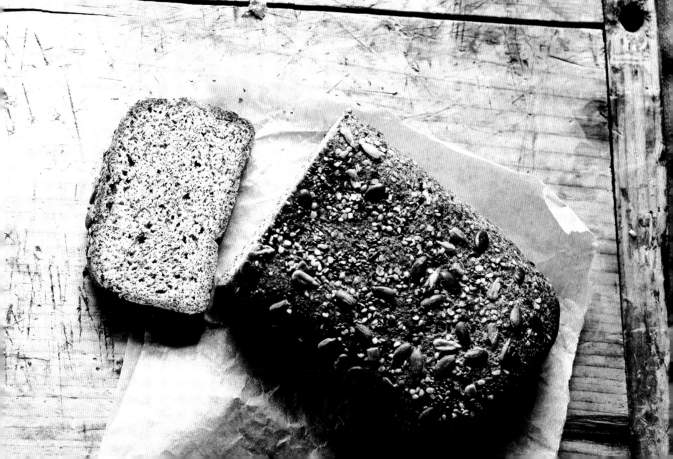

The biggest change in low-carb baking compared to traditional baking is that wheat flour, in fact any starchy flour, and sugar are firmly off the ingredients list as they raise your glucose levels and won't help weight loss.

Instead, here are a few new hero ingredients that will help your low-carb baking:

Psyllium husks – Found in health food shops and online, these are a form of insoluble fibre from the ovata plant, which works as a binder and helps baked goods rise. Buy blonde psyllium husks for golden bread and try to find the husks rather than the expensive powdered psyllium. This does work but can produce a purple colour in the bread. One word of warning, the psyllium husk needs to cool down after it is baked, as it firms up as it cools, so no nibbling on the bread before it is at room temperature, or you will find a soggy dough consistency. Regrinding the husks in a small high-speed food processor, though not essential, helps prevent a slimy texture to the bread.

Coconut flour – A fine powder that is very absorbent, so use in small quantities. It helps bind but also offers a natural sweetness to bread and pastry.

Mozzarella – Its job is to melt between the ingredients, holding them together and then to set firm on cooling. It leaves a mild savoury taste rather than a cheesy one. It's fine to use the inexpensive pizza mozzarella or the cow's milk one in a bag in the recipes in this chapter. Freeze any that is not used.

Ground almonds – The main substitute for wheat flour is finely ground blanched almonds, also known as almond flour in the US. You can grind your own almonds with or without the skin – the only difference is the colour. Almonds are low in carbs, high in fibre, have little flavour and add body and fat to baked goods.

Xanthan gum – Used in small quantities as a binder, thickener and emulsifier.

Arrowroot – Lower in carbs than cornflour, it is light and excellent at giving strength to dough as well as thickening sauces.

Golden flaxseed – Also known as linseed, it is cheaper to buy the whole seed and grind your own. The golden coloured seeds give a golden coloured bread and the darker seeds give an appearance of dark rye bread. The flavour is the same. Grind the seeds twice in a small high-speed food processor to make flour. Grinding it twice helps prevent a slimy texture to the bread. Flaxseed also helps to keep you regular and offers a good supply of omega 3 oil.

Butter – Usually it doesn't matter if it is salted or unsalted but try to always go for one made with milk from grass-fed cows.

Eggs – It doesn't matter if they are medium or large, but either extreme, i.e., very small or very large, might affect the result. I have added the size if it is important.

Seeds – High in protein and very nutritious. They can be used whole to add texture or ground to a flour as in the Super seed crackers recipe on page 73.

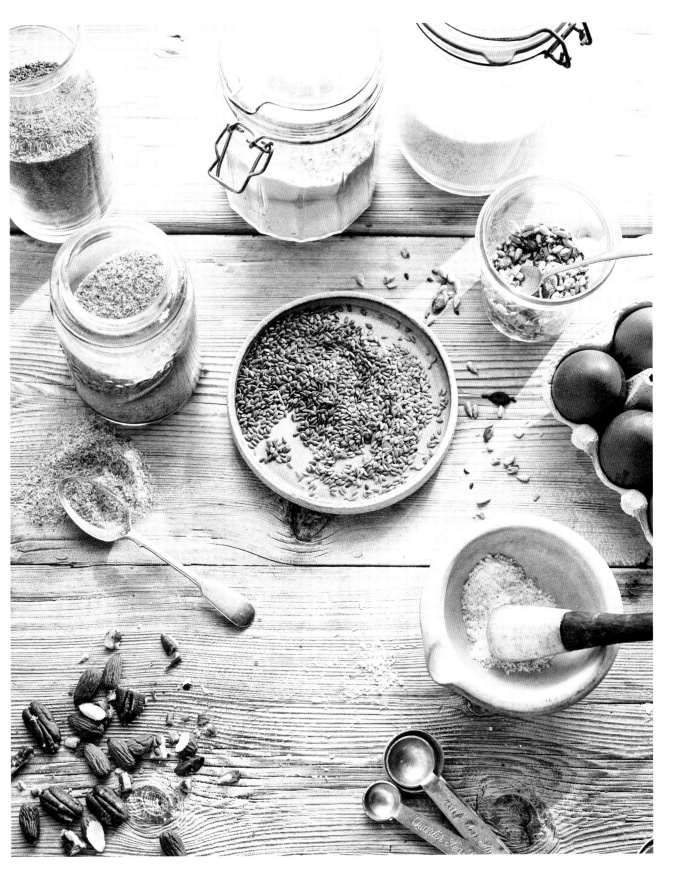

COUNTRY-STYLE LOAF

L

MAKES 16 SLICES

125g (4½oz) mozzarella, drained, torn into pieces

3 eggs

150g (5½oz) ground almonds

1 heaped teaspoon salt

2 teaspoons baking powder

80g (2¾oz) flaxseed, ground (use golden flaxseed for a lighter loaf)

25g (1oz) psyllium husks

200ml (7fl oz) cold water

extra virgin olive oil, for greasing

1 tablespoon seeds, such as sunflower, poppy or pumpkin (optional)

Per slice
1.1g net carbs, 3.9g fibre,
10g protein, 6.4g fat, 132kcal

I have had many readers ask me for a low-carb loaf they can cut into slices for sandwiches, so after much experimentation over the years, here is my sliced brown bread loaf! I have also given the method for making this into a country-style loaf which looks gorgeous but is harder to cut into even-sized slices.

Psyllium husk works as a binder to help the dough hold the rise without gluten and is available in all good health food shops and online. We prefer the husks of psyllium, not the superfine powder, which is more expensive. It will work in the same way but can produce a purple colour in your bread. You will notice there is mozzarella in the dough; you can use the inexpensive pizza mozzarella, and freeze any left over, as it grates more easily (though the soft ball of mozzarella works too).

To make the dough, put all the ingredients except the oil and seeds into a food processor and whizz until they form a ball of dough. If you prefer to make the dough by hand, grate the mozzarella into a bowl and combine with the remaining ingredients.

Preheat the oven to 220°C/200°C fan/425°F/gas mark 7.

To make the bread in a tin, line a 900g (2lb) loaf tin lengthways with a piece of baking parchment cut long enough so that you have a flap either side that hangs over the long edges. This will make it easier to remove the loaf. Brush the short sides of the tin with a little oil; there is no need to line them. Put the dough in the tin and press it down. Press on the seeds, if using.

To make the country-style loaf, lightly grease a baking tray with a little oil. Remove the dough from the food processor and put it on a lightly oiled work surface. Lightly oil your hands and mould the dough into a ball. Transfer it to the prepared baking tray and flatten the top a little so that you have a round loaf measuring about 15 x 5cm (6 x 2in). Scatter over the seeds, if using, and press them in. Cut a cross into the top using a serrated knife, making 2 slashes about 2cm (¾in) deep.

Bake either shaped loaf for 1 hour or until firm to the touch. Remove from the oven and leave to cool on a wire rack (out of the tin, if using) – don't cut it until it reaches room temperature.

Use the sliced bread as it is for a sandwich, or toast it. The loaf will keep in a sealed bag for 2 days out of the fridge or for 5 days in the fridge. The bread also freezes well (slice it first for easy defrosting) and will keep frozen for up to 3 months.

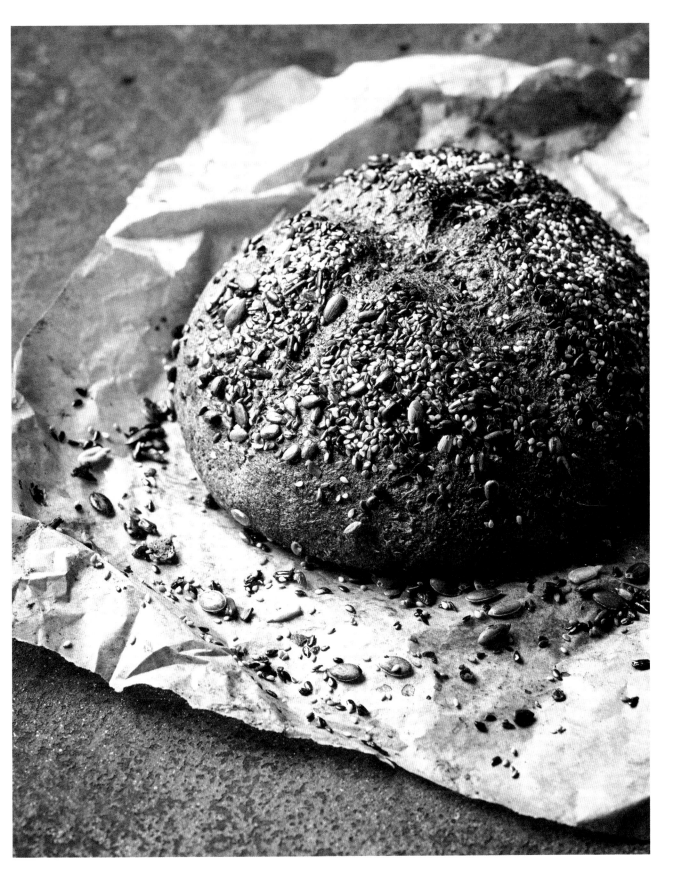

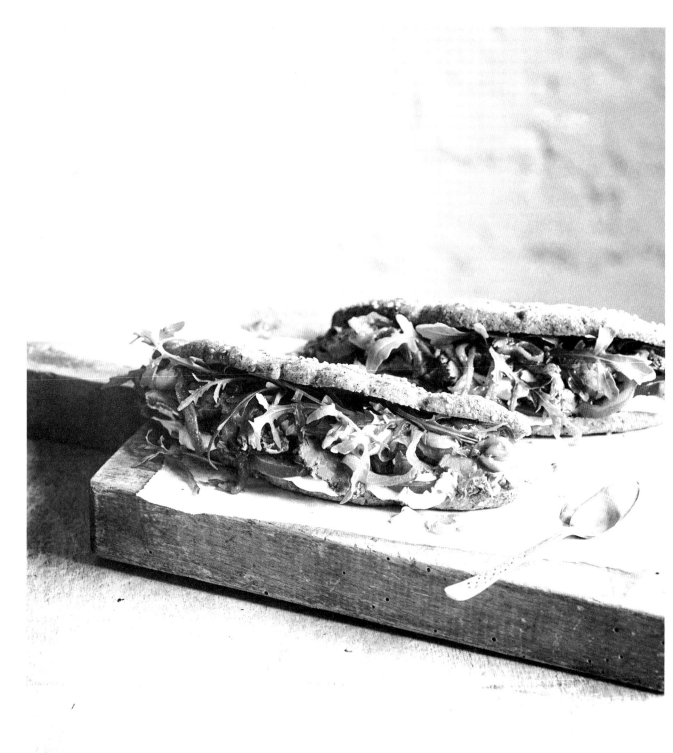

BROWN BREAD BAGUETTES

L

MAKES 2 SHALLOW BAGUETTES

olive oil, for greasing
30g (1oz) ground almonds
25g (1oz) psyllium husks
1 teaspoon baking powder
¼ teaspoon fine salt
2 medium or large eggs
beaten egg, for brushing (optional)
1 teaspoon sesame seeds (optional)

Per roll
2.1g net carbs, 11.5g fibre,
9.3g protein, 13.6g fat, 220kcal

While we normally suggest that a great big sandwich isn't a good idea, as the starches in the bread will raise your blood glucose levels, this is not the case with these low-carb baguettes. Your average 50g (1¾oz) bread roll contains about 30g net carbs, these contain just over 2g. This easy recipe is ideal for making rolls, bread for toasting and sandwiches. You can also make them in a batch and freeze them for quick meals. They defrost quickly in a microwave or warm place. Fill them with low-carb fillings such as ham, cheese, canned fish, leftover cooked meat with mayo or reheated roasted vegetables and mozzarella. And for a gorgeous, indulgent supper, try them as a steak sandwich (see page 68). You can prepare the filling as the rolls cook.

Preheat the oven to 220°C/200°C fan/425°F/gas mark 7 and grease a baking tray with a little oil.

Use a large metal spoon to mix the dry ingredients together in a mixing bowl. Then add the eggs and stir again until well blended.

Lightly wet your hands and use them to bring the dough into a ball. Divide the dough in half and hold one half between your hands, as if in prayer position, and press it into a short baguette with slightly pointed ends. Lay it down on the prepared baking tray and press gently into a long, flat, lozenge shape. It should be about 18 x 6 x 1 cm (7 x 2½ x ½in). Repeat with the remaining half of dough. The rolls are supposed to be flat as they are all about the filling, but you can mould them into whatever shape you like, if a round roll or even square suits you better.

Brush the rolls with beaten egg and scatter over the sesame seeds, if using.

Bake for 12 minutes or until golden brown and firm to the touch. Remove from the oven and leave to cool for at least 5 minutes. Cut carefully in half using a serrated bread knife, add your chosen filling and enjoy! The rolls will keep in a container or bag for 2 days out of the fridge or for up to 4 days in the fridge. They can also be frozen for up to 3 months.

STEAK SANDWICH

MAKES 2

1 tablespoon extra virgin olive oil
1 tablespoon butter
1 small onion, sliced into half-moons
150g (5½oz) fillet steak tails
2 Brown bread baguettes (page 67)
2 tablespoons mayonnaise
2 teaspoons Dijon or English mustard
1 tomato, sliced
a handful of rocket or 4 lettuce leaves
salt and freshly ground black pepper

Per steak sandwich
7.3g net carbs, 13g fibre,
26.5g protein, 35.8g fat, 511kcal

Fillet steak makes the perfect filling for a sandwich, as you can bite into it easily. By buying the fillet tails at the butcher's counter you will save on the cost. Use the baguettes on page 67. Serve with Dijon mustard or the One-minute mayonnaise on page 179. I like to add watercress, rocket or lettuce to my steak sandwich.

Heat the oil and butter in a medium frying pan until foaming. Add the onion and some seasoning and cook over a medium–high heat for about 10 minutes until soft and browned.

Meanwhile, put the fillet steak between 2 pieces of baking parchment or plastic (I use leftover florist's cellophane from a bunch of flowers) and bash the steak out to a thickness of 7mm (⅜in). You can use a meat tenderizer or the flat bottom of a small pan to do this. Season the steak on both sides.

Lift the onions into a bowl with tongs and keep in a warm place. Keep the pan.

Spread the rolls with the mayonnaise and mustard on both sides. Lay the tomato slices on the bottom halves and season with salt and pepper.

Heat the pan that you used to cook the onions over a medium–high heat. Put the steaks into the pan (one at a time if too big) and cook them for about 30 seconds or until just browned. Remove the steaks from the pan and cut into strips. Add the steak strips and the onions to the rolls, top with the rocket and put the tops on. Press down a little and cut each sandwich in half; serve straight away (with napkins for the juices!).

WHITE BREAD ROLLS

L   (depending on filling)
MAKES 8 BREAD ROLLS

olive oil, for greasing

75g (2¾oz) golden flaxseed, ground

100g (3½oz) ground almonds

2 teaspoons baking powder

½–1 teaspoon salt (depending on whether you use the mozzarella brine)

125g (4½oz) soft cow's milk or pizza mozzarella

75ml (2½fl oz) mozzarella brine from the bag or water

2 eggs, beaten

Per roll
1.2g net carbs, 4.3g fibre, 9.7g protein, 16g fat, 193kcal

This dough makes a white, light bread roll that is perfect for filling, making bacon rolls, toasting or splitting in half and using for open sandwiches. The rolls have a delicate flavour and are good for savoury or sweet toppings, despite containing mozzarella, which in this recipe acts as a binder. Instead of throwing the brine from a bag of mozzarella away, I like to use it in place of any additional water. If you do use the mozzarella brine, just add ½ teaspoon of salt.

Preheat the oven to 220°C/200°C fan/425°F/gas mark 7 and grease a baking tray with a little oil.

To make the dough, put all the ingredients into a food processor and whizz until they form a ball of dough. If you prefer to make the dough by hand, mix the dry ingredients together in a large bowl. Coarsely grate the soft mozzarella or finely grate the firm mozzarella by hand into the bowl. Add the mozzarella brine or water and eggs, then use a large spoon to mix everything together vigorously. You shouldn't be able to see any shreds of mozzarella in the dough.

Use a spoon to transfer 8 large spoonfuls of the dough to the prepared baking tray, placed at least 4cm (1½in) apart. I do this by putting 8 small mounds down and then dividing the remaining dough evenly between them.

Bake for 15–20 minutes or until golden brown and firm to the touch. Allow to cool to room temperature on a rack.

The rolls will keep in a container or bag for 2 days out of the fridge or for up to 4 days in the fridge. They can also be frozen for up to 3 months.

EASY PIZZA

MAKES 2 X 15CM (6IN) PIZZAS

For the pizza base

40g (1½oz) firm pizza mozzarella, finely grated

20g (¾oz) mature Cheddar or Parmesan cheese, finely grated

1 egg

50g (1¾oz) ground almonds or milled flaxseed

½ teaspoon baking powder

For the tomato sauce

40g (1½oz) tomato passata or puréed canned tomatoes

½ teaspoon dried oregano

¼ teaspoon salt

For the topping

50g (1¾oz) mozzarella, drained

2 teaspoons extra virgin olive oil

a few basil leaves

Further toppings (optional)

8 olives, pitted

4 canned sardines

1 teaspoon capers

a pinch of chilli flakes or sliced chilli, to taste

8–10 slices of salami

8 anchovies, drained from oil

Per pizza with tomato sauce, mozzarella, salami and olives
5.8g net carbs, 3g fibre, 22g protein, 39g fat, 479kcal

Each low-carb cookbook I have written contains a different pizza base. I like them all, but I know readers have their favourites. This recipe is based on the Fathead dough made famous by the movie of the same name (about low-carb eating and worth watching). And before Fathead, the recipe was created by Cooky Creations, who came up with the idea of using mozzarella in the pizza dough as well as on top. Genius, as it works as a binder and sets to a tearable cheesy crust.

You can use pizza mozzarella (the cheap one in a block) for the base, as it is easier to grate. It can also be used for the topping, but the best combination is pizza mozzarella for the base and a good full-fat cow's milk mozzarella for the topping. Any leftovers of each can be used for the White bread rolls or the Country-style loaf (see pages 69 and 64) or frozen. (Buffalo milk mozzarella is too watery for a pizza topping.) The pizza bases can be frozen and kept for up to 3 months.

These are small but filling pizzas but be happy; you are getting to eat gorgeous pizza and lose weight, so enjoy it and pile your plate with salad. To make the pizza bases nut free, use flaxseed instead of the ground almonds. And do try the sardine topping; it's so good, especially with anchovies and chilli.

Preheat the oven to 220°C/200°C fan/425°F/gas mark 7 and line a baking tray with baking parchment.

Put all the ingredients for the pizza base together in a bowl and mix with a large metal spoon. It will form a thick, sticky dough.

Divide the dough in half and transfer to the prepared baking tray. Press and shape each half with wet hands into a 15cm (6in) circle about 1cm (½in) deep. Bake for 6 minutes or until firm to the touch and lightly brown.

Meanwhile, mix the tomato sauce ingredients together in a small bowl.

Remove the tray from the oven. (At this stage the bases can also be cooled, wrapped tightly in clingfilm and kept in the fridge for 3 days or frozen for 3 months. Defrost before use.)

Top each pizza base with half the tomato sauce, using the back of a spoon, and leaving a finger-width border around the edge. Tear over the mozzarella and add your chosen toppings. Bake for 5 minutes until the mozzarella is bubbling and the crust is crisp and browned. Remove from the oven and serve with a drizzle of oil and scattered with the basil leaves.

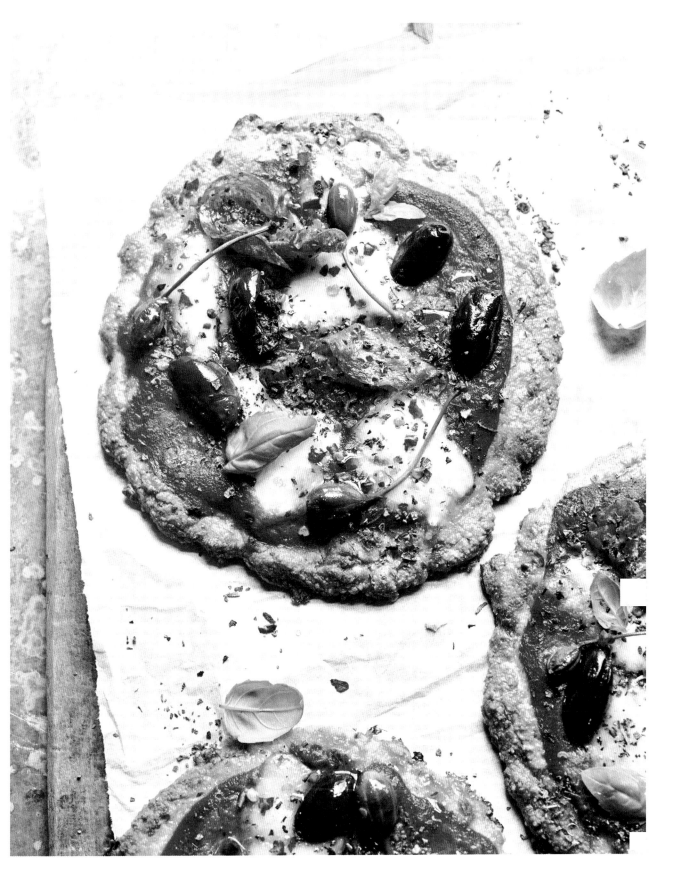

SAUSAGE ROLLS

L

MAKES 12

6 high-meat-content sausages or
    400g (14oz) sausage meat

1 egg yolk, beaten, to glaze

1 tablespoon sesame seeds
    (optional)

For the pastry

130g (4½oz) ground almonds

½ teaspoon xanthan gum

1 teaspoon baking powder

pinch of salt

30g (1oz) butter or lard, softened

1 egg

Per serving (2 rolls)
2.8g net carbs, 2.6g fibre,
9.4g protein, 22.4g fat, 260kcal

Rather than smothering sausage rolls in tomato ketchup, mustard is a sugar-free option. Xanthan gum gives strength to low-carb pastry. Try to find high-meat-content sausages containing no rusk or flour, to keep the carbs down.

Preheat the oven to 200°C/180°C fan/400°F/gas mark 6 and cut 2 pieces of baking parchment the same size as a large baking tray.

Use a large metal spoon to mix the dry ingredients together for the pastry. Add the butter and egg and mix to form a smooth, well-blended dough. If your pastry is very dry, which can happen if your egg is small, add 1 tablespoon of water to help it bind together. Use your hands to gather it into a ball and remove it from the bowl. Divide the pastry in half and gently roll each half into a sausage shape.

Place the dough sausages on one piece of baking parchment about 10cm (4in) apart. Lay the other piece of baking parchment on top and roll the dough into 2 long, thin rectangles. Cut and move pieces of pastry to form 2 rectangles about 30 x 12cm (12 x 4½in) and 3mm (⅛in) thick.

Peel the skin from the sausages (or squeeze the meat out) and lay 3 along the centre of each of the dough rectangles. Some sausages are shorter or fatter than others, but you can squeeze or stretch the sausage meat out to fit the length. Use the parchment to roll up the dough to cover the sausages. Trim the edges as necessary. Cut each roll into 6 pieces. Use one piece of baking parchment to line the baking tray. Lift the sausage rolls on to the prepared tray and brush with the egg yolk. Scatter over the sesame seeds, if using. Bake for 20 minutes until the pastry is golden brown.

Serve warm or at room temperature. Once cooled, they will keep in a container in the fridge for up to 3 days or freeze for up to 3 months.

VEGGIE ROLLS

50g (1¾oz) rolled oats

150g (5½oz) beetroot, coarsely grated

100g (3½oz) feta cheese,
    coarsely grated

1 large egg

1 heaped teaspoon ground cumin

pinch of salt

Whizz the oats in a food processor until they resemble sand. Mix the oats with the remaining ingredients in a large bowl, using a large spatula, until well blended. Lightly wet your hands and roll the mixture into a long sausage shape. Use this instead of the sausages to fill the sausage rolls and follow the recipe as above.

Per serving (2 rolls)
7.8g net carbs, 3.4g fibre, 10.2g protein, 22.2g fat, 282kcal

SUPER SEED CRACKERS

U

SERVES 8

extra virgin olive oil, for greasing

150g (5½oz) mixed seeds, such as
    sunflower, pumpkin, poppy, hemp,
    coriander or sesame

1 teaspoon fine salt

1 egg white

1 tablespoon black onion
    (nigella) seeds

Per serving 30g (1oz)
3.4g net carbs, 0.5g fibre,
4.5g protein, 8.5g fat, 109kcal

Make your own low-carb, gluten-free seed flour easily at home by grinding seeds in a small food processor or using a stick blender. The crackers can also be left plain without the onion seeds, or you can add cumin or caraway seeds instead. Once the crackers are bone dry, they will keep in a paper bag at room temperature for a week. These are lovely with butter and cheese or Giorgio's moutabal (page 148) and tomatoes.

Preheat the oven to 180°C/160°C fan/350°F/gas mark 4, line a baking tray with baking parchment and lightly brush it with oil.

Grind the mixed seeds (not including the black onion seeds) into a coarse flour in a small food processor or using a stick blender.

Mix the seed flour with the salt and egg white in a large mixing bowl and add 100ml (3½fl oz) cold water. Thoroughly mix the ingredients together to form a thick paste. Use a spatula to scrape the mixture on to the prepared tray.

Take another piece of baking parchment the size of your baking tray and brush it with oil. Put this, oil-side down, on top of the mixture and use your hands to push the mixture evenly over the base to a thickness of 2mm (⅟₁₆in). Slowly peel away the top sheet of parchment and scatter over the black onion seeds. Put the parchment back over the top and press down to seal in the seeds.

Remove the top piece of parchment again and bake for 25–30 minutes or until lightly browned and brittle.

Once cool enough to touch, break the crackers into shards or use a knife to cut them. If any of the crackers look undercooked underneath, simply put them back in the oven for a couple of minutes to crisp up.

PROVENÇAL-STYLE TART WITH SMOKED SALMON, CRÈME FRAÎCHE & CHIVES

L
SERVES 6

For the pastry

175g (6oz) ground almonds

25g (1oz) Parmesan cheese, finely grated

½ teaspoon xanthan gum

1 teaspoon baking powder

¼ teaspoon salt

30g (1oz) butter or lard, softened

1 egg

For the filling

150ml (5fl oz) soured cream or crème fraîche

1 large egg

150g (5½oz) smoked salmon, roughly torn

a small handful of chives, finely sliced

a large handful of rocket leaves

salt and freshly ground black pepper

This makes a delicious pastry that is easy to work with, doesn't need to be rested and can be topped with a creamy filling and whatever you have in the fridge. I often substitute the salmon and chives for goat's cheese and thyme for vegetarian friends.

Preheat the oven to 220°C/200°C fan/425°F/gas mark 7 and cut 2 pieces of baking parchment to fit your oven tray.

To make the pastry, put all the ingredients into a mixing bowl with 2 tablespoons of water and use a metal spoon to mix them together thoroughly. Use your hands to bring the mixture into a ball.

Transfer the pastry to one of the pieces of baking parchment. Put the other piece over the top and roll out the pastry to form a rectangle measuring about 32 x 23cm (12¾ x 9in); it will be about 5mm (¼in) thick. Don't worry if you need to cut off pieces and replace them to achieve a rectangle. Peel off the top sheet of parchment.

Slide the parchment and pastry on to the oven tray. Use the parchment to fold the edges in on themselves to make a 1cm (½in) raised border around the outside to trap in the filling.

Mix the soured cream and egg together and season with salt and pepper. Pour this mixture into the pastry tart and scatter over the salmon and chives. Bake for 15 minutes or until golden brown on the edges and top. Serve hot, warm or at room temperature topped with the rocket.

Per serving
3.2g net carbs, 4.2g fibre,
18g protein, 31g fat, 371kcal

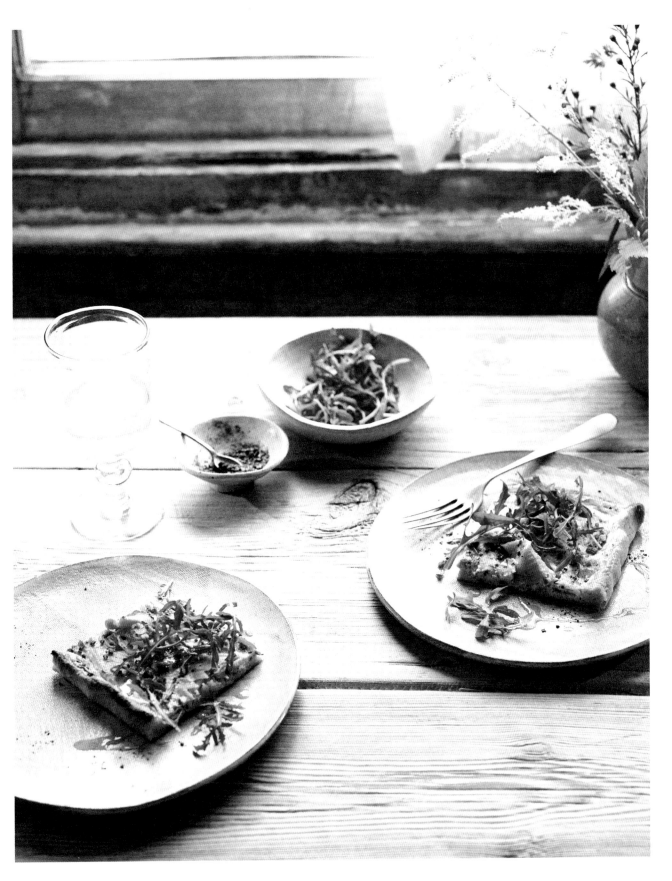

CLASSIC CHICKEN & LEEK PIE

SERVES 8

1 egg yolk, beaten, to glaze

For the pastry

150g (5½oz) cold salted butter,
 cut into small cubes

200g (7oz) ground almonds

30g (1oz) coconut flour

1 medium egg

For the filling

850g (1lb 14oz) cooked chicken
 breast, diced

75g (2¾oz) reserved chicken fat,
 olive oil, ghee or butter

400g (14oz) trimmed leeks, split in
 half lengthways and washed,
 then cut into 2cm (¾in) pieces

2 bay leaves

½ teaspoon grated nutmeg

4 tablespoons cornflour

750ml (1⅓ pints) whole milk

salt and plenty of freshly ground
 black pepper

Per serving

16g net carbs, 5.8g fibre,
38g protein, 43g fat, 614kcal

This family favourite is now back on the menu with our buttery, crumbly low-carb pastry and creamy chicken and leek filling. I have taught this recipe plenty of times on my Zoom courses and people are always amazed at how easy the pastry is to make. Use leftover turkey instead of chicken after Christmas or use half ham and half chicken to change things up.

Cut 2 pieces of baking parchment 5cm (2in) larger than your pie dish, which should measure about 25cm (10in) square.

To make the pastry, use a food processor or your fingers to blend the butter with the ground almonds and coconut flour in a bowl. Make sure it is well combined and there are no lumps of butter remaining. Add the egg and use a spoon or the food processor to mix it in. Scrape the pastry into a ball and lay it in the centre of one of the pieces of baking parchment, flatten lightly and wrap up. Rest in the fridge while you make the filling.

Fry the chicken in the fat in a large frying pan over a medium–high heat, scattered with a little salt, until browned all over. Use a slotted spoon to transfer the chicken to the pie dish and set aside.

Set the pan back over a medium heat and fry the leeks in the remaining fat, with a splash of water, covered, for about 10 minutes or until just soft, turning occasionally. Remove the lid and add the bay leaves, nutmeg, salt and pepper and scatter over the cornflour. Cook for a minute, stirring through, then add the milk. Bring to the boil, stirring continuously for a few minutes until the sauce has thickened. Taste and adjust the seasoning. Remove the bay leaves and pour the sauce over the chicken, then stir through and set aside. Leave to cool for 15 minutes.

Preheat the oven to 190°C/170°C fan/375°F/gas mark 5.

Unwrap the pastry and sandwich it between the 2 pieces of parchment. Roll it out so that it is about 4mm (¼in) thick and large enough to cover your pie dish. (Hold the pastry between the sheets of baking parchment over the dish to check.) Peel off the top sheet of parchment and then turn the pastry and the bottom sheet of parchment on to the pie. Don't worry if it cracks, just push the pastry together and into place. Trim off the excess and use a fork to seal the edges. Use any leftover pastry as decoration if you like. Brush the top of the pastry with beaten egg yolk and make a hole in the centre to let the steam out of the pie. Bake for 25–30 minutes or until golden brown. Serve with any green vegetables you like.

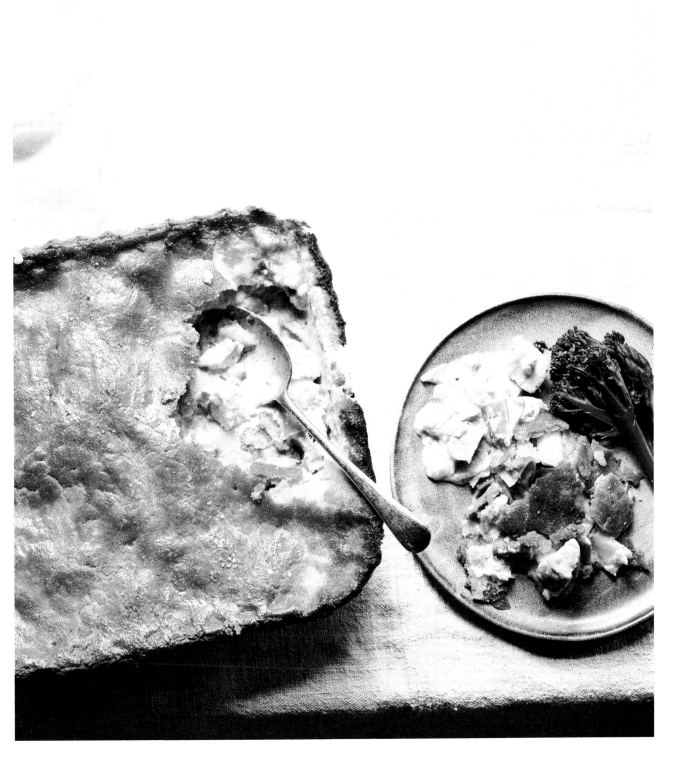

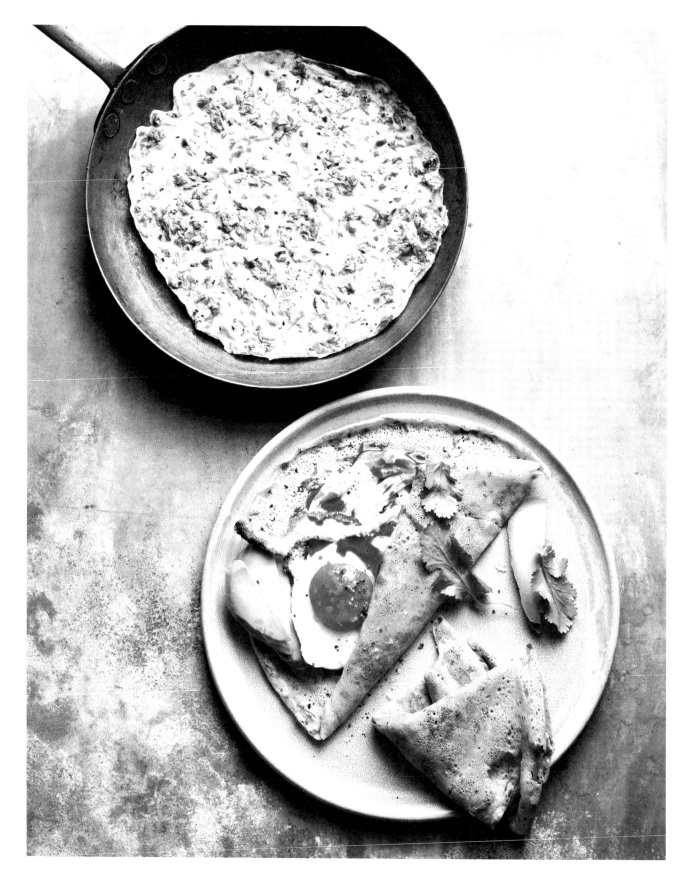

COCONUT CRÊPES

L

MAKES 10 CRÊPES APPROX.
16CM (6¼IN)

35g (1¼oz) coconut flour

50g (1¾oz) arrowroot

2 eggs

1 teaspoon black onion (nigella) seeds

½ teaspoon salt

coconut oil or ghee, for frying

Added extras (optional)

a small handful of coriander, finely chopped

1 tablespoon black onion (nigella) seeds

1 tablespoon cumin seeds

1 teaspoon sesame seeds (optional)

Per serving
8.3g net carbs, 2.5g fibre,
14g protein, 16g fat, 244kcal

I love how thin yet strong these crêpes are and how you can use them for sweet or savoury dishes. This recipe is inspired by Lauren Geertsen and her brilliant blog Empowered Sustenance. My addition is to use herbs and seeds in the batter. Coriander leaves and black onion (nigella) seeds are probably my favourite. I have a stack of these crêpes in a bag in the fridge so we can quickly fry an egg and make a fast, light meal. They will keep in the fridge for up to 4 days and freeze for up to 3 months. Arrowroot can be used to thicken sauces and is more widely available these days. In this recipe it binds the ingredients together and gives strength to the crêpes for easy flipping, filling and wrapping.

Make the batter by whisking all the ingredients, except the coconut oil, together with 350ml (12fl oz) water in a bowl. Whisk in any added extras, if you are using them, now too. The batter should be the consistency of double cream. If it is too watery, add a teaspoon or two of coconut flour to absorb the liquid or add more water if it doesn't swirl around the pan sufficiently. Keep the whisk in the bowl and give it a stir between crêpes.

Choose your best medium non-stick frying pan and put over a medium–high heat. Add a small knob of coconut oil and brush this over the base of the pan with a silicone pastry brush or a piece of folded kitchen paper.

When you can feel the heat on your palm above the pan, pour 3 tablespoons of the batter into it and swirl the pan around to form a circular crêpe about 16cm (6¼in) across. Be patient! Wait for the pancake to be cooked underneath before you attempt to flip it. It will start to curl at the edges and release itself from the pan.

Use a fish slice or spatula to release the crêpe from the pan and flip it over or toss it in the air to turn. Cook the other side until lightly brown. They will take about 4 minutes; be prepared to increase and reduce the heat so that they cook quickly but don't burn. Wipe the pan between crêpes. You will soon get the hang of using your pan, adjusting the heat and flipping.

As the crêpes are cooked, stack them on a plate. They can be eaten warm or at room temperature. They will keep in the fridge for up to 4 days and freeze for up to 3 months.

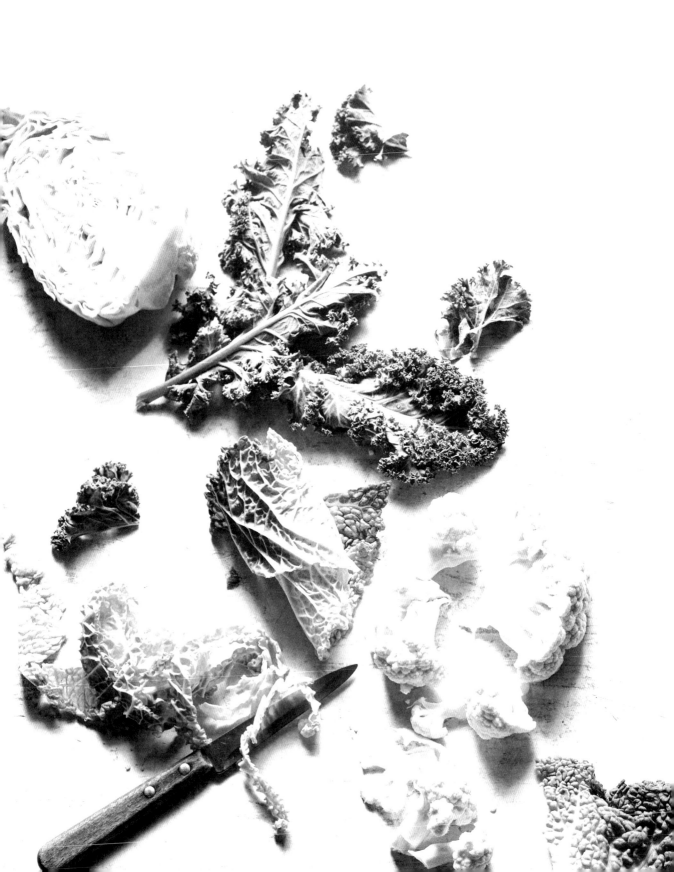

CARB
CRUSHERS

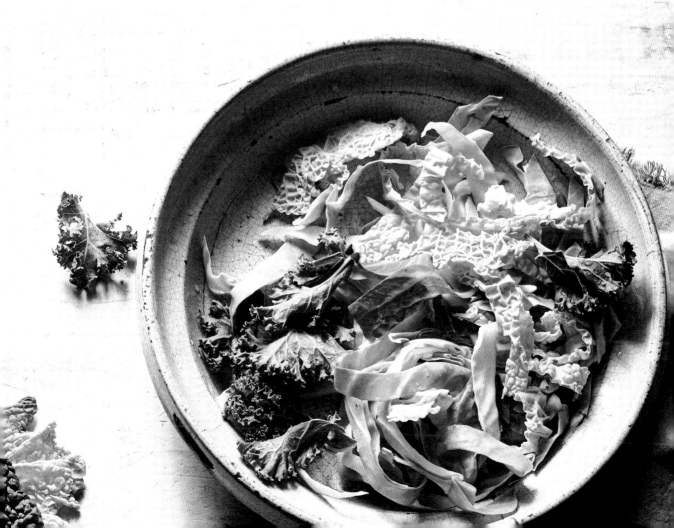

SPINACH & RICOTTA GNUDI IN SAGE BUTTER

MAKES 36/SERVES 4 AS A MAIN

For the gnudi

300g (10½oz) squeezed-dry spinach

250g (9oz) ricotta

50g (1¾oz) Parmesan cheese, grated

50g (1¾oz) mature Cheddar cheese,
    coarsely grated

2 large eggs

60g (2¼oz) coconut flour

½ teaspoon finely grated nutmeg

salt and freshly ground black pepper

For the sauce

100g (3½oz) butter

12 medium sage leaves

30g (1oz) toasted pine nuts (optional)

25g (1oz) Parmesan cheese,
    finely grated

Per serving
of gnudi
10.6g net carbs, 8.1g fibre,
19.4g protein, 19.3g fat, 321kcal

of gnudi in sauce
12.4g net carbs, 8.1g fibre,
22.3g protein, 46.2g fat, 574kcal

Gnudi, pronounced "neudi", means "nude" referring to the naked filling of spinach and ricotta ravioli without their pasta clothes. Traditionally they are served in a warm bath of sage-flavoured butter but gnudi are equally good in a ragù or tomato sauce. Frozen spinach is fine to use but do buy whole-leaf and not chopped spinach. My other tip is to squeeze the spinach three times; you will be amazed how much water comes out of it and, be warned, it will ruin the gnudi if it is still wet. You can use your hands to squeeze the spinach or try squeezing balls of it between two plates. Frozen spinach doesn't need to be cooked, only defrosted. Incidentally a 900g (2lb) bag of frozen whole-leaf spinach gives you about 300g (10½oz) once squeezed dry. To get that amount from fresh spinach, you need about 600g (1lb 5oz).

To make the gnudi, finely chop the squeezed-dry spinach by hand or pop it into a food processor and briefly blitz it. Then mix all the ingredients together in a large mixing bowl until well combined. It should form a thick paste; if it is very sticky, add a spoonful of coconut flour to absorb the moisture. If you know how to make quenelles (a shape similar to a rugby ball), form these out using 2 dessertspoons. Alternatively, use your hands to roll the mixture into walnut-sized balls and set them aside on a plate or two.

Prepare the sauce by melting the butter in a large frying pan. Add the sage leaves and some salt and pepper (if using) and fry until the leaves are lightly browned. Add a ladleful of hot water and stir well. Pour half the sauce into a warm serving jug and leave the remaining half in the pan over a very low heat while you cook the gnudi.

Bring a large pan of well-salted water to the boil. Reduce the heat to medium – you want a slow rolling, not rapid, boil. Drop the gnudi gently into the boiling water. Let the water come back up to the boil and cook the gnudi for 3–4 minutes until they rise up to the surface. Let them bob around for a further minute, then remove them from the water with a slotted spoon and lower them gently into the butter sauce in the pan. Fry the gnudi gently for a couple of minutes. This helps set the outside and lightly browns them.

Add the reserved sauce to the pan and the pine nuts, if using. Divide between bowls and serve topped with the grated Parmesan.

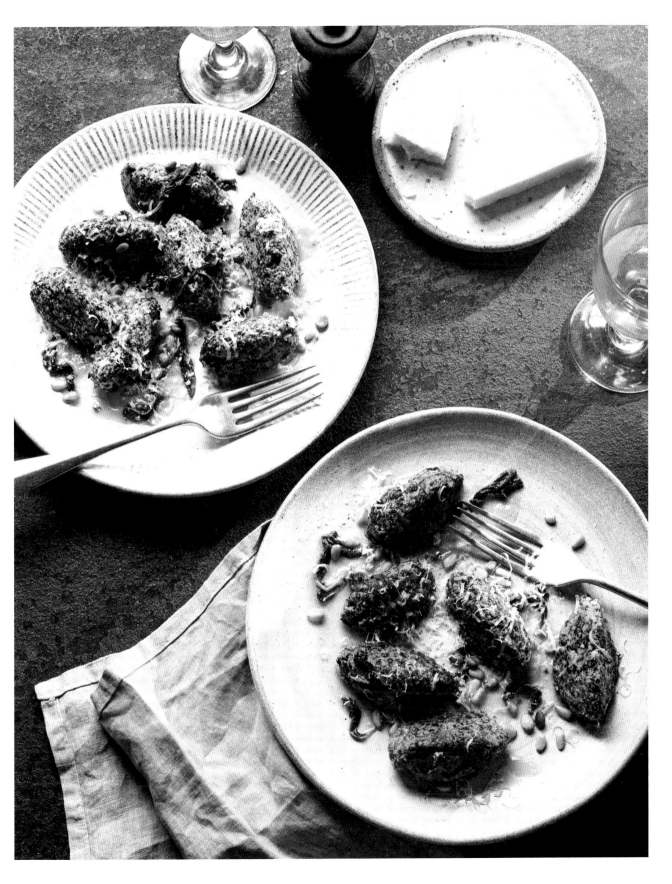

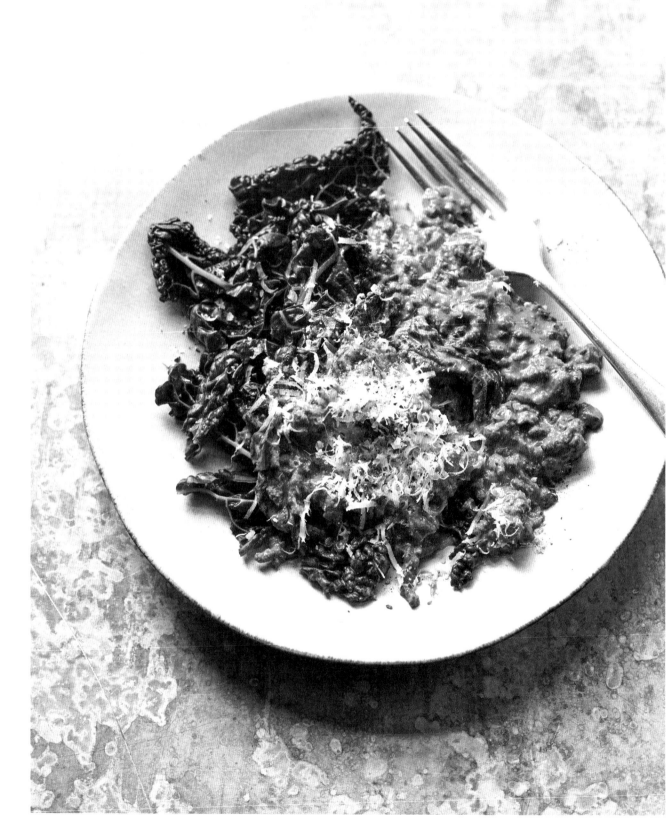

BOLOGNESE RAGÙ ON KALE PEZZI

SERVES 8

6 tablespoons extra virgin olive oil

1 red or white onion, finely chopped

1 medium carrot, finely chopped

1 celery stick, finely chopped

600g (1lb 5oz) beef mince
(preferably 15% fat)

200g (7oz) pancetta or unsmoked
streaky bacon, minced in a food
processor or cut finely by hand

200g (7oz) chicken livers,
finely chopped

400ml (14fl oz) red wine

2 x 400g (14oz) cans of Italian
plum tomatoes

200ml (7fl oz) warm meat stock
or hot water

100ml (3½fl oz) double cream

salt and freshly ground black pepper

15g (¼oz) Parmesan, finely grated,
to serve

For the kale pezzi (Serves 2)

300g (10½oz) cavolo nero

Per serving
of ragù and cheese
10.5g net carbs, 3.2g fibre,
25g protein, 29.3g fat, 450kcal

of kale pezzi
1g net carbs, 2.8g fibre,
2.4g protein, 1.1g fat, 122kcal

On a mission to find the perfect Bolognese sauce many years ago, I once ate ten bowls of it over three days in Bologna, all delicious and all quite different from one another in their ingredients and the shape of the pieces of meat (no wonder I needed a low-carb diet!). Further research and speaking to as many Bolognese as possible led me to conclude that there is no definitive recipe. Most include chicken livers and pancetta, which make the ragù really rich in flavour. I was shown how to soften and meld the flavours together with milk, but to keep the carbs down we use cream here instead. Don't be tempted to use smoked pancetta or bacon because it will completely dominate the dish.

Cut the onion, carrot and celery into very small cubes or briefly whizz them in a food processor. Frying them first gives a wonderful base flavour to the dish and is called a *soffritto*. The dark, slightly bitter leaves of cavolo nero (black kale) are softened by the sweet and spicy sauce in this delicious combination but any cabbage will work. We have torn the kale into pieces or *pezzi* in Italian. The sauce keeps well for 5 days in the fridge and freezes well too.

Heat the oil in a heavy-based saucepan over a medium–high heat. Add the onion, carrot, celery and some salt and pepper. Once they start to sizzle, reduce the heat to medium and fry them gently for 12–15 minutes until softened.

Add the mince, pancetta and chicken livers and fry for 10–15 minutes over a medium–high heat, stirring frequently and breaking up the meat until the water has been released and evaporated. The mixture should be sizzling and sound dry as it is stirred.

Add the wine and cook over a high heat for 5 minutes until the wine has separated from the oil. At this point, add the tomatoes, rinsing out the cans with the stock, and add this too. Bring the ragù to the boil, then reduce the heat to a simmer and cook for 2 hours. Stir through the cream and cook for a further 30 minutes. Adjust the seasoning to taste. The Bolognese ragù is now ready to serve or to cool and store.

To make the kale pezzi, strip the leaves from the stems of the cavolo nero and tear them into pieces about 5cm (2in) wide. Discard the stems. Wash the leaves and put them into a saucepan of boiling lightly salted water for about 5 minutes or until tender.

Reheat 2 portions of the Bolognese ragù in a frying pan. Drain the leaves and mix with the sauce or put the sauce on top of the cavolo nero, scatter over the Parmesan and serve.

GIORGIO'S 'NDUJA & MUSHROOM SAUCE

SERVES 2

200g (7oz) mushrooms, sliced

2 tablespoons extra virgin olive oil

1 garlic clove, peeled and lightly
crushed with the flat side of a knife

1 small white onion, thinly sliced
into half-moons

10 cherry tomatoes, halved

3 tablespoons 'nduja or
cooking chorizo

a pinch of chilli flakes (optional)

For the roast sprouts

300g (10½oz) Brussels sprouts,
trimmed and halved, or quartered
if large

2 tablespoons extra virgin olive oil
or beef or chicken dripping

a few sprigs of thyme or rosemary
or 1 teaspoon dried thyme

15g (½oz) Pecorino or Parmesan
cheese, finely grated

salt and freshly ground black pepper

Per serving
of 'nduja and mushroom sauce
6.5g net carbs, 2.2g fibre,
10.7g protein, 19.7g fat, 243kcal

of roasted sprouts and cheese
6.8g net carbs, 3.9g fibre,
5.9g protein, 16.3g fat, 200kcal

'Nduja is a soft, spicy sausage from Calabria in southern Italy. You can find it in delis, large supermarkets or online. Our son Giorgio loves it on everything from the Coconut crêpes on page 79 rolled up with a fried egg, to Hot buttered toast on page 51 and stirred into sauces. It adds a wonderful spicy depth of flavour to everything it touches. You could use soft cooking chorizo instead. Roasting Brussels sprouts brings out the flavour and gives them a lovely texture. They are gorgeous as a side or as a substitute for short pasta such as penne.

Preheat the oven to 200°C/180°C fan/400°F/gas mark 6.

Toss the sprouts in the olive oil in a bowl with the herbs and some seasoning, then lay them on a roasting tray in a single layer and roast for 15–20 minutes or until lightly browned and just soft.

Heat a large frying pan over a medium–high heat and add the mushrooms. Dry-fry them, stirring frequently for 7–10 minutes, until they have lost the water and started to brown, then add the oil, garlic and onion and continue to cook for 5–7 minutes until the onion has softened.

Add the cherry tomatoes and 'nduja to the pan and stir through. Let the 'nduja melt and tomatoes soften, then taste the sauce. As brands of 'nduja differ you may need a little salt or more chilli to taste.

Transfer the sprouts to 2 warm bowls and pour over the 'nduja sauce. Scatter over the Pecorino and serve.

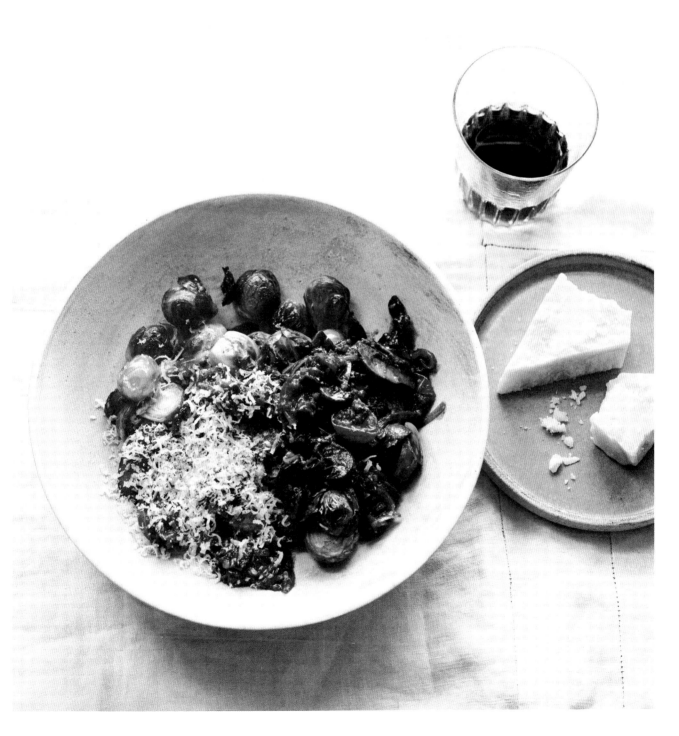

CABBAGE RIBBONS, MUSHROOMS & PARMESAN CREAM

SERVES 2

For the mushrooms

250g (9oz) chestnut or wild
mushrooms, sliced

2 garlic cloves, peeled

2 tablespoons extra virgin olive oil

a few sprigs of thyme or rosemary,
finely chopped, plus extra to serve

For the cabbage ribbons

300g (10½oz) Savoy, sweetheart or
other cabbage

20g (¾oz) salted butter or olive oil

salt and freshly ground black pepper

For the Parmesan cream

30g (1oz) mature hard cheese
such as Parmesan, Manchego
or Pecorino, finely grated

75ml (2½fl oz) double cream

Per serving
of mushrooms and Parmesan cream
4g net carbs, 1.5g fibre,
8.5g protein, 38g fat, 392kcal

of cabbage ribbons
4.5g net carbs, 4.7g fibre,
3.1g protein, 5.9g fat, 91kcal

There are three parts to this recipe but don't let that put you off. Each stage is very simple and can be used independently. The cabbage ribbons go with any pasta sauce or are wonderful as a side dish. Use any cabbage to make the ribbons but allow longer for thicker leaves, such as white cabbage, to cook. The Parmesan cream is about the easiest cheese sauce you can make and can be used over steamed cauliflower as a quick cauliflower cheese or to make cheesy leeks. And finally, the mushrooms are simply sautéed and are gorgeous as a side dish or over a Chaffle for breakfast (see page 44). To bump up the protein, add a poached egg to the finished dish and for extra decadence add a swirl of truffle oil just before serving.

Heat a large frying pan over a medium–high heat and add the mushrooms. Dry-fry them, stirring frequently, for 5–7 minutes until the water comes out of them and they start to brown. Lightly crush the garlic cloves with the flat of a knife, add them to the pan with the oil and herbs and cook for a couple of minutes until you can smell them. Remove the pan from the heat.

To make the cabbage ribbons, remove any damaged, outer leaves from the cabbage. Now pull away the next few leaves and cut out the triangle of hard core. Check now that you have the correct weight of these trimmed cabbage leaves. (Since I don't like to waste food, I finely slice the pieces of core and use in a salad or add them to the ribbons.) Roll up the leaves, two at a time, and cut them into ribbons similar in width to tagliatelle. Put the cabbage ribbons into a medium saucepan with the butter, 4 tablespoons of water and some seasoning and cover with a lid. Cook over a medium heat for 5 minutes or until it is tender.

To make the Parmesan cream, heat the cheese and cream together in a small pan over a very low heat for 5 minutes, stirring frequently. Use straight away if you need a runny cream or continue to heat until it reduces and thickens to your liking. Serve directly from the pan or leave to cool and reheat later as you need it.

Reheat the mushrooms in the pan. Drain the cabbage from the water as soon as it is ready and tip it into the mushroom mixture with a little of the cooking water. Toss through and serve in warm bowls drizzled with the cheese sauce and scattered with thyme or rosemary.

GREEN BEANGUINE ALL'AMATRICIANA

SERVES 6

5 tablespoons extra virgin olive oil

500g (1lb 2oz) onion, finely sliced into half-moons

250g (9oz) guanciale, pancetta or streaky bacon, cut into 5mm (¼in) strips

100ml (3½fl oz) white wine

2 × 400g (14oz) cans of Italian plum tomatoes

salt and freshly ground black pepper

For the green beanguine (Serves 2)

280g (10oz) green, runner or flat beans

a knob of butter

15g (½oz) Pecorino Romano or Parmesan cheese, finely grated

Per serving
of sauce
9.9g net carbs, 3.7g fibre,
8.3g protein, 30.5g fat, 364kcal

of beanguine and cheese
6.6g net carbs, 4.5g fibre,
4.8g protein, 6.5g fat, 111kcal

The world-famous tomato and onion sauce, Amatriciana, comes from Amatrice, a town in the mountainous region of Lazio. This area was Abruzzo before Mussolini changed the border lines. The mountain people who lived there called the sauce *la gricia*, which was simply fried guanciale, black pepper, Pecorino and sometimes vinegar. Tomatoes were a later addition by the wealthier people of the area who could afford them, and it then became known as amatriciana.

Guanciale, or cured pig's cheeks, is the background meaty flavour imparted by the layers of fat and meat in a cheek that has been coated in pepper and hung in a curing cabinet for months. This renders the guanciale sweet, firm to slice and with a kick of umami that is not delivered by mass-produced bacon. If you can't find this, or pancetta, buy pancetta lardons or the best unsmoked streaky, fatty bacon you can find.

The sauce makes enough for 6 portions, but it keeps in the fridge for up to 5 days and can be frozen for up to 3 months.

Heat the olive oil in a large frying pan and add the onion, guanciale, a pinch of salt and a generous amount of pepper. Fry over a medium heat for about 15 minutes until the onion has until completely softened.

Add the wine and allow to reduce for about 5 minutes, then add the tomatoes. Use a potato masher to crush the tomatoes to a rough pulp and gently simmer for 30 minutes until the sauce reduces and thickens. Taste and add more seasoning as necessary.

Meanwhile, prepare the beans. Green beans should be topped but the tails can be left intact. Either leave them long or cut the beans into short lengths like penne pasta if you find that easier to eat. String and slice runner and flat beans into long lengths using a vegetable peeler, sharp knife or bean slicer. Put the beans into a small saucepan with the butter, a pinch of salt and 3 tablespoons of water. Cover with a lid and cook over a medium heat for 5–8 minutes or until soft and no longer squeaky. Remove the lid and set aside.

Reheat 2 portions of the sauce in a frying pan. Drain the beans and mix with the sauce or put the sauce on top of the beans, scatter over the cheese and serve.

CLASSIC ITALIAN TOMATO SAUCE WITH BROCCOLI ALLA SORRENTINA

L
SERVES 6

For the classic Italian tomato sauce

5 tablespoons extra virgin olive oil

1 red onion, finely chopped

1 garlic clove, lightly crushed

1 teaspoon salt

2 x 400g (14oz) cans of Italian
  plum tomatoes

freshly ground black pepper

For the broccoli alla Sorrentina (Serves 2)

125g (4½oz) mozzarella

400g (14oz) broccoli florets

⅓ x quantity Classic Italian
  tomato sauce

a handful of basil leaves

15g (½oz) Parmesan or Pecorino
  cheese, finely grated

Per serving
of classic Italian tomato sauce
6.9g net carbs, 1.3g fibre,
1.8g protein, 11g fat, 139kcal

of broccoli alla Sorrentina with classic
Italian tomato sauce
13g net carbs, 6.9g fibre,
22g protein, 26g fat, 393kcal

This is a classic baked pasta dish from Sorrento on the Amalfi coast of Italy. It is normally made with potato gnocchi, but we have substituted carby potatoes for bite-sized broccoli. The tomato sauce contains no sugar, so if you weren't going super low carb and wanted to have this on pasta then you would still be eating more healthily than using a sugar-loaded commercial brand of pasta sauce. Next time you are at the supermarket about to buy a jar of tomato sauce, just have a look at the ingredients – nearly all versions contain sugar, which simply isn't necessary in a good Italian tomato sauce.

This tomato sauce recipe serves 6 and keeps in the fridge for up to 5 days or can be frozen. You can use it over the Italian roast vegetables on page 174 or with the Mighty meatloaf on page 118. The Broccoli alla Sorrentina serves two but you can double or triple the recipe as necessary.

To make the sauce, heat the olive oil in a saucepan over a medium heat and fry the onion and garlic for 7–10 minutes until softened and translucent. Season with the salt and some pepper.

Add the tomatoes and rinse the cans out with a little water, then add this to the pan too. Bash the tomatoes with a potato masher or wooden spoon to break them up. Reduce the heat and simmer, uncovered, for about 40 minutes to concentrate the flavours. The sauce should be thick and not watery. Taste and adjust the seasoning as necessary.

Tear the mozzarella into about 10 pieces and put into a sieve over a bowl to get rid of any water. Cut the broccoli into bite-sized florets and cook in a saucepan of boiling salted water for about 5 minutes or until the stalks are just tender. Drain and set aside.

Heat the grill to high.

Put the broccoli into an ovenproof dish and pour over the tomato sauce. Scatter over half the basil leaves, the mozzarella and Parmesan. Put the dish under the grill for 8–10 minutes or until the cheese is golden brown and bubbling. Serve topped with the remaining basil leaves.

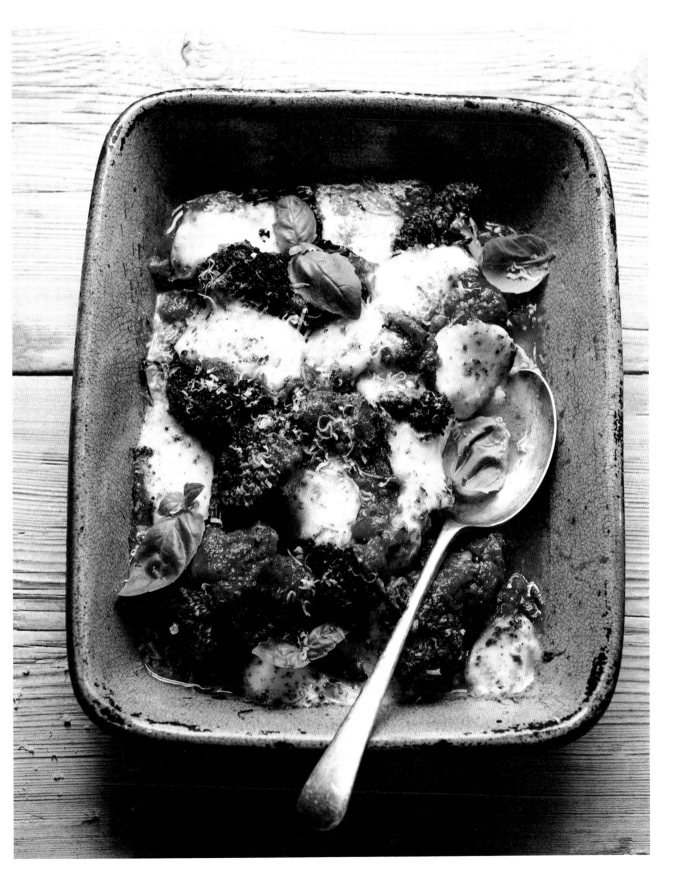

CHAPATTIS

L

MAKES 10 CHAPATTIS APPROX.
14CM (5½IN)

100g (3½oz) tablespoons coconut
    flour

50g (1¾oz) golden flaxseed, ground

2 tablespoons psyllium husks

1 teaspoon salt (optional)

1 teaspoon baking powder

1 tablespoon cumin, black onion
    (nigella), sesame or coriander
    seeds (optional)

a knob of ghee or coconut oil,
    for frying

Per chapatti
3.4g net carbs, 6g fibre, 3.4g protein,
4.3g fat, 85kcal

After much experimentation, I am really happy with this low-carb dough which can be rolled thin enough to use as a chapatti or all-purpose wrap. This recipe also has the advantage of being vegan, nut-free and gluten-free. We love the flavour and natural sweetness that the coconut brings to the party. I prefer the warm colour of golden flaxseed but if you only have the dark brown variety, it will do just fine. Do use psyllium husks and not the powdered version if possible.

The chapattis can be rolled out and neatly cut into circles or left with ragged edges as you like. Enjoy them plain, salted, speckled with seeds or simply slathered in melting ghee.

Mix the dry ingredients together in a bowl with a large metal spoon and add 325–350ml (11–12fl oz) water a little at a time. When the spoon is useless, use your hands to mix everything into a dough, then set aside for 5 minutes to allow the water to be absorbed.

Heat a non-stick frying pan over a medium–high heat.

Divide the dough into 10 pieces and roll each one between your palms to form a walnut-sized ball (about 50g/1¾oz). Now roll each dough ball between 2 pieces of baking parchment with a rolling pin to a thickness of about 2mm (1/16in). You can put a 14cm (5½in) saucer or pan lid on to the dough and cut around it for neat, circular chapattis or leave them with ragged edges as you like.

Add a knob of ghee or coconut oil to the pan and swirl the pan so the oil coats the base – you only need a light covering. (If your pan is very non-stick, you may not need any oil, or you might need a little more oil to cook the chapattis if the pan isn't at all non-stick.)

Peel a chapatti off the parchment and lay in the pan. Cook for 3 minutes on each side, depending on the heat, until well browned and cooked through. Roll the next chapatti as the first cooks, then add to the pan. Repeat with the remaining dough. You can use a spatula to flip the chapattis and to remove them from the pan as they are ready.

Serve the chapattis warm or at room temperature. They will keep, covered, in the fridge for 5 days or for 3 days out of the fridge. They freeze well for up to 3 months.

CAULI RICE

U
SERVES 4

approx. 600g (1lb 5oz) cauliflower
  (flower, stalk and leaves)

3 tablespoons extra virgin olive oil,
  ghee, coconut oil, chicken fat or
  beef dripping

1 onion, finely chopped, or 5 spring
  onions, finely chopped

salt and freshly ground black pepper

Per serving
5.8g net carbs, 3.3g fibre,
3.1g protein, 10.6g fat, 134kcal

I think this is the best method of making cauli rice, shown to me by our friend Sally Dorling. It takes just minutes to prepare; leave it as it is or embellish it with herbs or spices as you stir-fry it. It keeps well in the fridge for up to 3 days once cooked (or in the freezer for up to 3 months). You can also use broccoli or sprouts in the same way.

Cut the head of cauliflower into large florets and roughly chop the stalk and leaves. Put a third of the cauliflower into a food processor and pulse until finely chopped (it will resemble large grains of rice), making sure you don't end up with a purée. Tip the cauliflower into a bowl and repeat with the remaining two thirds. If you don't have a food processor, coarsely grate the florets and stalk and finely chop the leaves.

Heat the fat in a wok or large frying pan. Fry the onion over a medium heat for 7 minutes or until soft. Add the cauliflower rice, season generously and stir through. Add 3 tablespoons of water, cover and leave to cook over a low heat for 5–7 minutes or until just soft, stirring occasionally. Taste and add seasoning as necessary. Serve straight away or leave to cool and reheat later. The rice will keep, cooked and cooled, in the fridge for up to 4 days. It can be reheated in a pan with a lid or in the microwave.

PILAO CAULI RICE

U
SERVES 4

2 garlic cloves, grated

10g (¼oz) fresh ginger, grated

pinch of chilli flakes, to taste

1 small cinnamon stick

4 split cardamom pods

½ teaspoon ground turmeric

salt and lots of freshly ground
  black pepper

a few sprigs of coriander,
  leaves picked and stems
  finely chopped

We love this with curries; however, it is a versatile dish that goes with pretty much everything.

Follow the recipe for Cauli rice (see above), adding the garlic, ginger, chilli flakes and spices when the onion has softened. Fry over a medium heat for 2 minutes, then follow the basic recipe. Stir in the coriander just before serving.

Per serving
6.8g net carbs, 3.4g fibre, 3.2g protein, 10g fat, 138kcal

CHORIZO & PEPPER CAULI RICE

SERVES 2

180g (6oz) cooking chorizo, sliced

1 small onion, finely sliced

1 small red pepper, roughly chopped

¼ teaspoon chilli flakes or a little
hot fresh chilli, to taste

2 garlic cloves, finely chopped
or crushed

2 tablespoons extra virgin olive oil

300g (10½oz) cauliflower, riced
(see page 93)

2 teaspoons harissa paste

5 tablespoons hot water

12 black olives, pitted, approx.
50g (1¾oz)

50g (1¾oz) feta cheese, crumbled

a handful of flat-leaf parsley,
stems finely chopped and
leaves roughly chopped

salt and freshly ground black pepper

Per serving
19g net carbs, 5.8g fibre,
25.3g protein, 40.2g fat, 555kcal

Y viva España! All the flavours of a Spanish holiday will be in your kitchen with this low-carb cheat's version of paella. It can be made in around 20 minutes and becomes a big bowl of vibrant taste and colour. Do try to find high-meat-content or preferably all-meat chorizo; you don't want ones stuffed with rusk and flour. For a vegetarian alternative, skip the chorizo and add a little more feta.

Fry the chorizo, if using, onion, red pepper, chilli and garlic in the oil in a large frying pan (for which you have a lid) over a medium–high heat. Add the cauli rice, harissa and hot water and stir through, then add the olives and bring to the boil. Reduce the heat, put on the lid and simmer for 6 minutes or until the cauliflower is soft. Remove the lid, taste and season as necessary. If any water remains, allow it to evaporate over a medium–high heat for a couple of minutes, stirring constantly.

Scatter over the crumbled feta and parsley and serve.

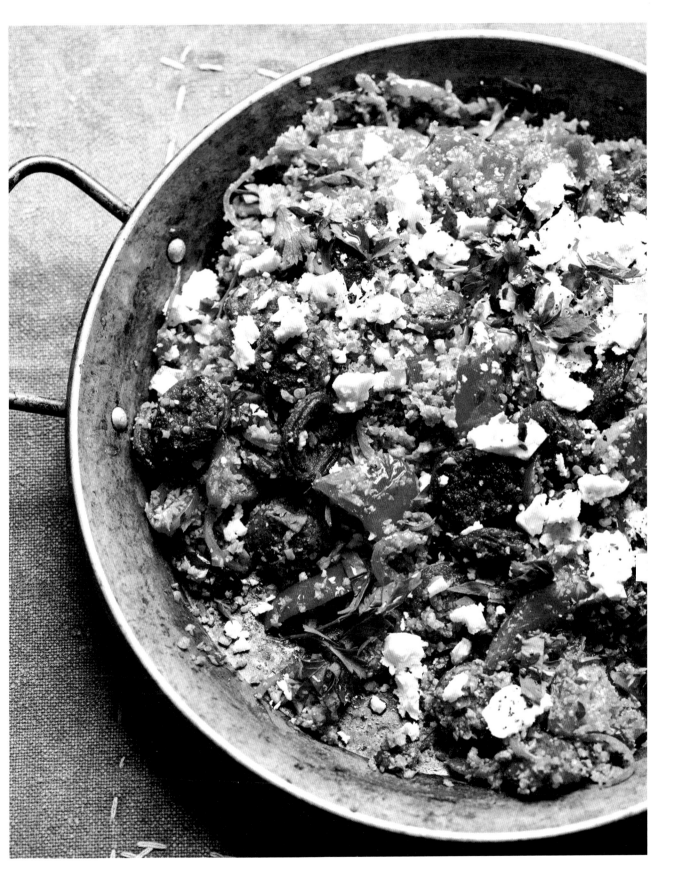

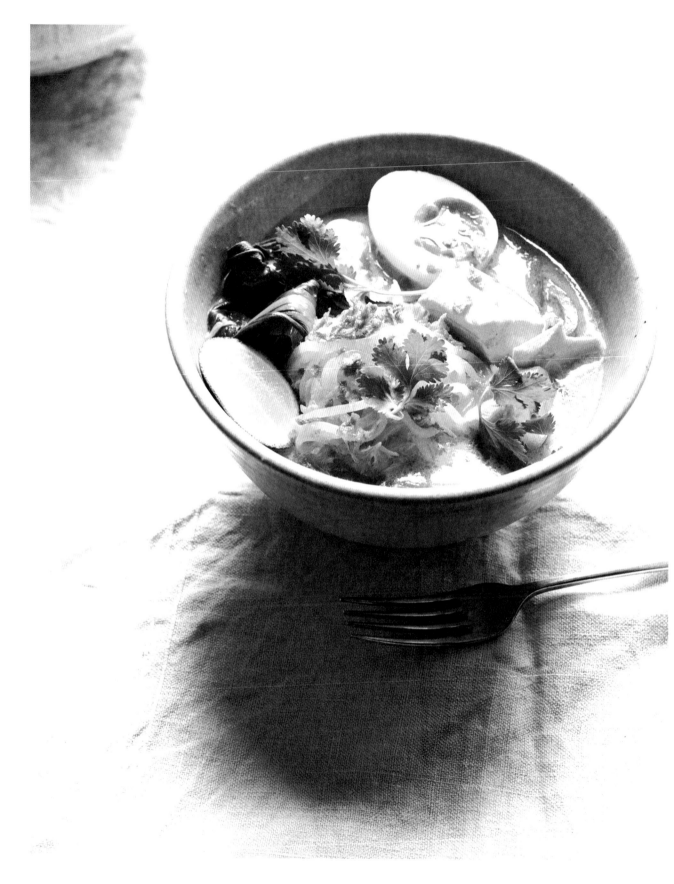

SALMON LAKSA

SERVES 4

For the spice paste

25g (1oz) fresh ginger, peeled

2 garlic cloves, peeled

2 small hot red chillies or more if you like it hotter

1 lemongrass stalk, tough outer leaf removed, roughly chopped

5cm (2in) piece of fresh turmeric, peeled, or ½ teaspoon ground turmeric

1 teaspoon salt

For the noodle soup

1 tablespoon coconut oil, ghee or extra virgin olive oil

1 banana shallot or 1 small onion, finely sliced

1 red pepper, thinly sliced

400ml (14fl oz) can of coconut milk

500ml (18fl oz) warm fish or chicken stock or water

2 fresh or dried lime leaves

2 pak choi or choi sum (approx. 175g/6oz), roughly chopped

600g (1lb 5oz) salmon, skinned and cut into 4cm (1½in) pieces

fish sauce (optional)

350–400g (12–14oz) konjac noodles

To serve

1 quantity of crispy onions from page 144 or shop-bought ones

4 soft-boiled eggs

a small handful of coriander (optional)

lime wedges

It is easy to make your own laksa spice paste if you have a small food processor or you don't mind chopping and pounding in a pestle and mortar. I like to make twice the amount and freeze half for another day. Alternatively, buy a good brand of ready-made laksa paste or Thai red curry paste. This recipe is loosely based on Cambodian chef Susie Jones' recipe. She told me there are so many ways to make Laksa, as this delicious bowl of spicy comfort is found all over South East Asia.

We have used salmon here, but Susie sometimes uses canned sardines or tuna, or adds boiled and shredded chicken instead of fish. To make the laksa vegan, use squares of tofu instead of the salmon and omit the fish sauce. You can buy zero-carb noodles, also known as konjac or shirataki noodles, in most supermarkets; they have been enjoyed in Japan for their texture for centuries. They are made from the konjac root and are a good source of insoluble fibre, so they make you feel full; they are very low in calories and have zero carbs.

Start by making the spice paste: blend the ginger, garlic, chillies, lemongrass and turmeric with the salt and 100ml (3½fl oz) water to a smooth paste in a mini food processor.

To make the noodle soup, heat a large saucepan over a low heat, add the coconut oil and fry the banana shallot for 7 minutes or until soft and translucent. Add the red pepper and stir-fry for a couple of minutes. Add the spice paste and stir-fry for a further couple of minutes until sizzling and fragrant.

Pour in the coconut milk, stock and lime leaves, bring to the boil, then reduce the heat and simmer gently, uncovered, for 5 minutes. Add the pak choi and simmer for a minute. Add the salmon and cook for about 5 minutes or until the fish is just cooked.

Taste the soup and adjust the flavour with salt and fish sauce to your liking.

Wash the noodles thoroughly in a sieve, then pour a kettle full of hot water over them. Divide the drained noodles between 4 warm, deep bowls. Ladle the laksa broth over the noodles. Top with the crispy onions, boiled eggs and coriander, if using, and serve with the lime wedges alongside.

Per serving
9.3g net carbs, 7.3g fibre, 46.8g protein, 35.1g fat, 568kcal

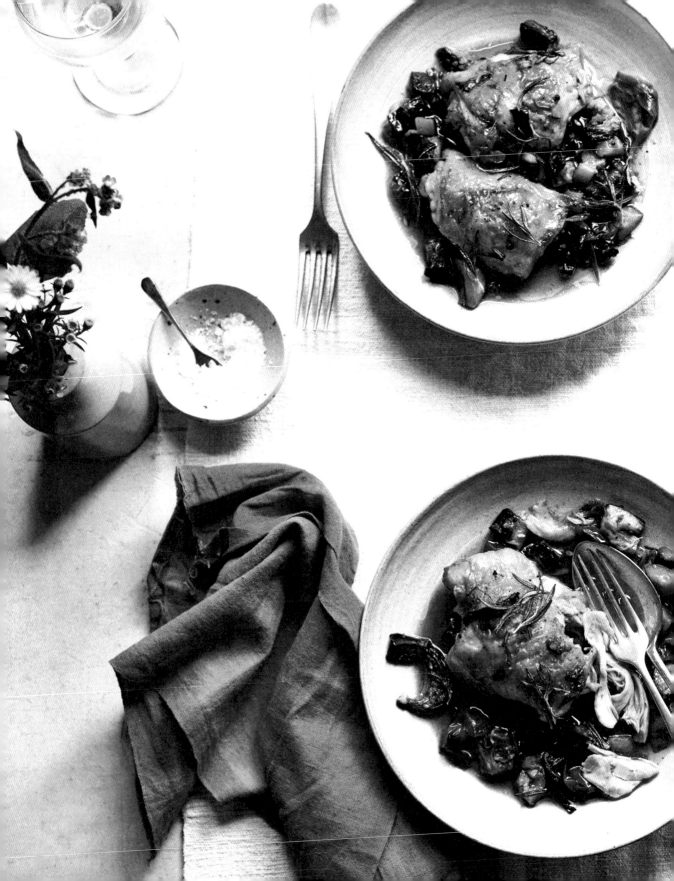

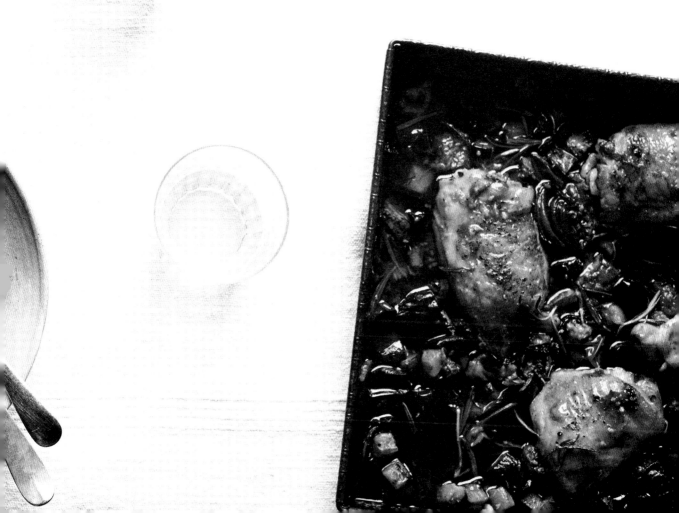

MEAT & POULTRY

YE OLDE POTTAGE

L

SERVES 4

3 tablespoons extra virgin olive oil,
  ghee or reserved chicken fat

250g (9oz) onions or leeks, or a
  mixture, finely chopped

1 medium carrot

2 celery sticks

250g (9oz) root vegetables, such
  as turnips, celeriac or parsnips,
  cut into 1cm (½in) dice

½ teaspoon salt and plenty of freshly
  ground black pepper

a few sprigs of thyme or 1 teaspoon
  dried thyme

1 large sprig of rosemary

a few sprigs of sage or 1 teaspoon
  dried sage

2 bay leaves

200g (7oz) leaves, such as cabbage,
  kale, sprouts, spinach or a mixture

1.2 litres (2 pints) chicken stock

250g (9oz) cooked chicken, turkey or
  gammon, roughly torn or
  chopped into bite-sized pieces

Per serving
6.5g net carbs, 5.6g fibre,
23g protein, 5.6g fat, 178kcal

Pottage is a wondrously thick and tasty soup which has been in existence since medieval times in Britain, hence the tongue-in-cheek recipe title. The ingredients depended on what was in season and were simply added to stock in a cauldron suspended over a fire. This makes four good bowls of soup but do double the batch for more portions as it freezes well and keeps for up to 4 days in the fridge.

This recipe is a perfect example of the continuous kitchen. A phrase meaning that one meal contributes to another; in this case, the stock made from a previous roast and the leftover dripping and meat make the soup. And the stock is key in this recipe. My best version of Pottage is always after picking the meat from the bones of the turkey after Christmas or Easter and making a stock from the carcass. The rest of the year I save my carcasses from roast chickens and make a batch of stock from those.

I find it quicker to chop and cook at the same time for this recipe. Heat the oil or fat in a large saucepan over a medium heat. Start by adding the onions while you finely chop the carrot and add that, followed by the chopped celery and root vegetables. Season with the salt and pepper, add the herbs and cook for 10 minutes, stirring frequently.

Roughly chop and add the leaves and stir through until they begin to wilt. Pour in the stock and bring to the boil. Reduce the heat so the soup is just bubbling and cook for 30 minutes or until the root vegetables are cooked through and tender.

Stir in the chicken and cook until it is heated through. Taste the pottage and add more seasoning if necessary. Serve hot.

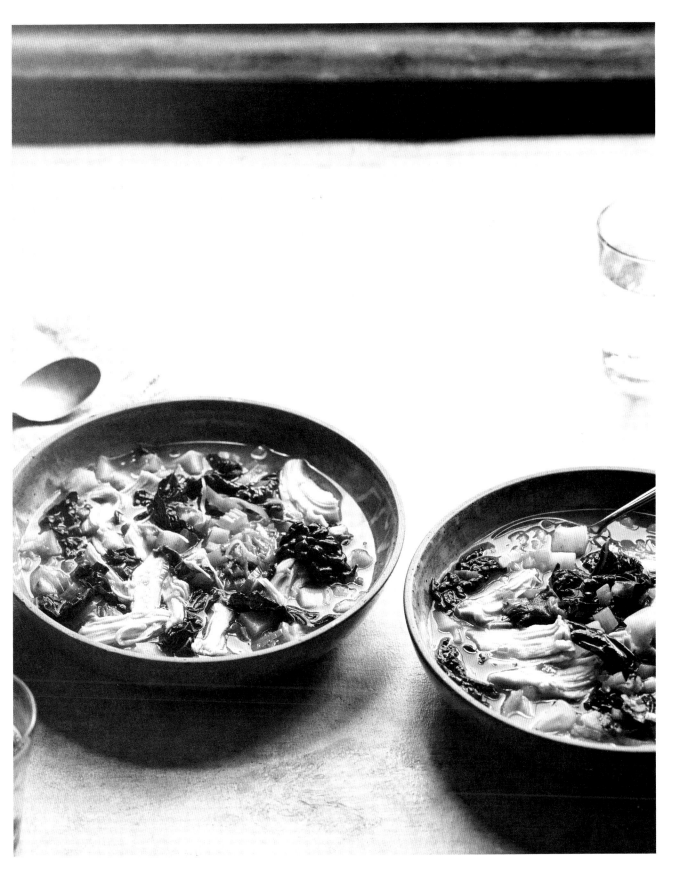

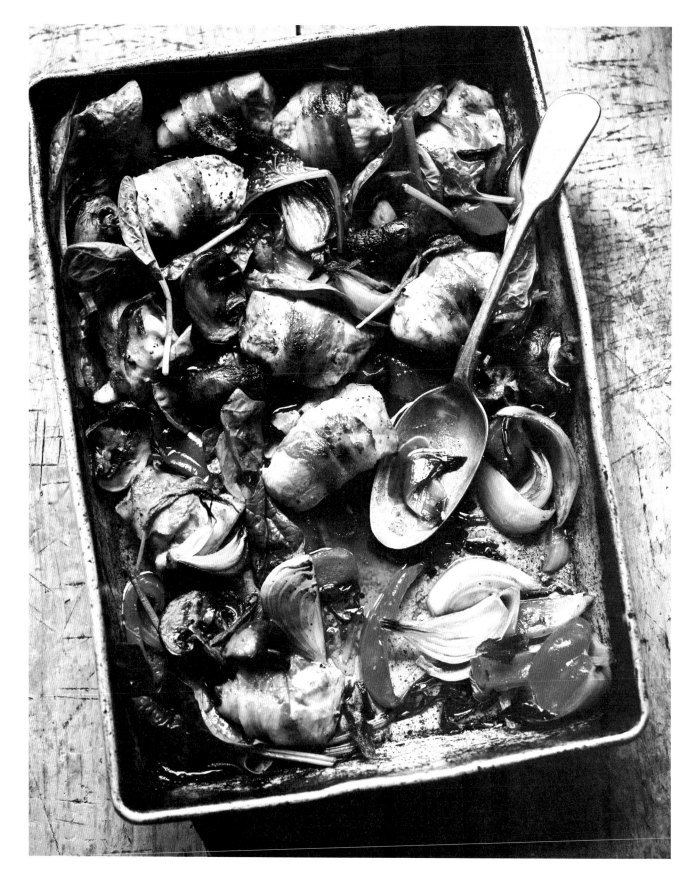

CHICKEN WRAPPED IN BACON

SERVES 4

4 medium (600g/1lb 5oz) skinless
    chicken breasts

16 rashers thinly cut, smoked streaky
    bacon (approx. 250g/9oz)

1 onion, roughly sliced into wedges

200g (7oz) chestnut or other
    mushrooms, halved

1 red pepper, cut into strips

12 sage leaves (optional) and/or
    4 rosemary sprigs

6 tablespoons extra virgin olive oil

2 tablespoons balsamic vinegar

100g (3½oz) baby spinach leaves

salt and freshly ground black pepper

Per serving
6.5g net carbs, 2.2g fibre,
59.3g protein, 42.2g fat, 653kcal

This quick crowd-pleaser was rustled up for us by Stefano Borella, chef and
teacher at our cookery school. Don't worry if you don't have any fresh herbs,
a sprinkling of dried oregano or thyme also does the trick. Serve as it is or
with a simple salad.

Preheat the oven to 240°C/220°C fan/475°F/gas mark 9.

Cut each chicken breast into four even-sized pieces. Wrap each piece
in one rasher of bacon and put them on a roasting tray. Add the onion,
mushrooms, red pepper and herbs to the tray. Scatter over a little
seasoning and pour over the oil and vinegar. Toss everything together
with your hands and tuck the herbs underneath.

Cook for 15–20 minutes until the chicken is cooked through. To test this, cut
into the thickest piece of chicken and see if it is pink inside. As long as it is
white all the way through, the chicken is done. Scatter over the spinach
and stir through. Serve straight away.

SIMPLE ROAST CHICKEN WITH MUSHROOM & CREAM SAUCE

Ⓖ with sides of your choice
SERVES 6

1.8kg (4lb) chicken

1 head of garlic, halved horizontally

a small handful of thyme sprigs,
    1 heaped teaspoon dried thyme
    or 3 sprigs of rosemary

50g (1¾oz) butter

150ml (5fl oz) dry white wine

salt and freshly ground black pepper

For the mushroom & cream sauce (optional)

500g (5½oz) chestnut mushrooms,
    halved if large

150ml (5fl oz) chicken stock or water

200g (7oz) crème fraîche

For the gravy (optional)

150ml (5fl oz) chicken stock or water

25g (1oz) butter

1 tablespoon arrowroot or cornflour

a squeeze of lemon juice (optional)

Per serving of chicken with mushroom & cream sauce
3.7g net carbs, 0.7g fibre,
29.5g protein, 32.6g fat, 447kcal

of chicken with gravy
3.6g net carbs, 0.2g fibre,
27.9g protein, 23.8g fat, 362kcal

This is very straightforward to make, and we love it with Sautéed greens and Celeriac mash (see pages 167 and 173). Do keep the leftovers for stock and the Ye olde pottage on page 100. I have given you the choice of making an easy creamy sauce with crème fraîche and mushrooms or a simple gravy. I thicken it with arrowroot as it is lower in carbs than cornflour, although that works just as well.

Preheat the oven to 200°C/180°C fan/400°F/gas mark 6.

Put the chicken into a roasting tin. Tuck the garlic halves under the chicken and put the thyme into the cavity. Use a knife to spread the butter evenly over the breast. Season all over with ¾ teaspoon of salt and some pepper.

Roast for 1 hour, then baste the bird with the cooking juices that have collected in the tin. Add the mushrooms around the edges, if you are making the mushroom and cream sauce, and toss to coat in the fat. Add a little more seasoning over the mushrooms, if using. Continue to cook for a further 30 minutes or until done.

Check the chicken is cooked through by inserting a temperature probe into the bird in the thickest part. It should be over 80°C (176°F). If you don't have one, insert a skewer into the thickest part of the bird, usually above the leg and into the breast. The juices that run out should be clear and not pink.

When you are happy that the chicken is cooked, remove the tin from the oven and use tongs or a large fork to hold the chicken upright over the tin to empty the cavity of juices. Pull out the thyme sprigs and add these to the roasting tin. Put the chicken on a warm or wooden carving dish and lightly cover with foil and a cloth to keep it warm. Leave it to rest for 20 minutes, this is really important to help keep the chicken juicy.

Put the tin over a medium heat. Add the white wine and bring to the boil. Scape off the brown bits from the bottom of the tray and squeeze out the garlic. Discard the skins and pick out the thyme stems. Let the wine reduce by half or until the strong smell of alcohol has turned sweet.

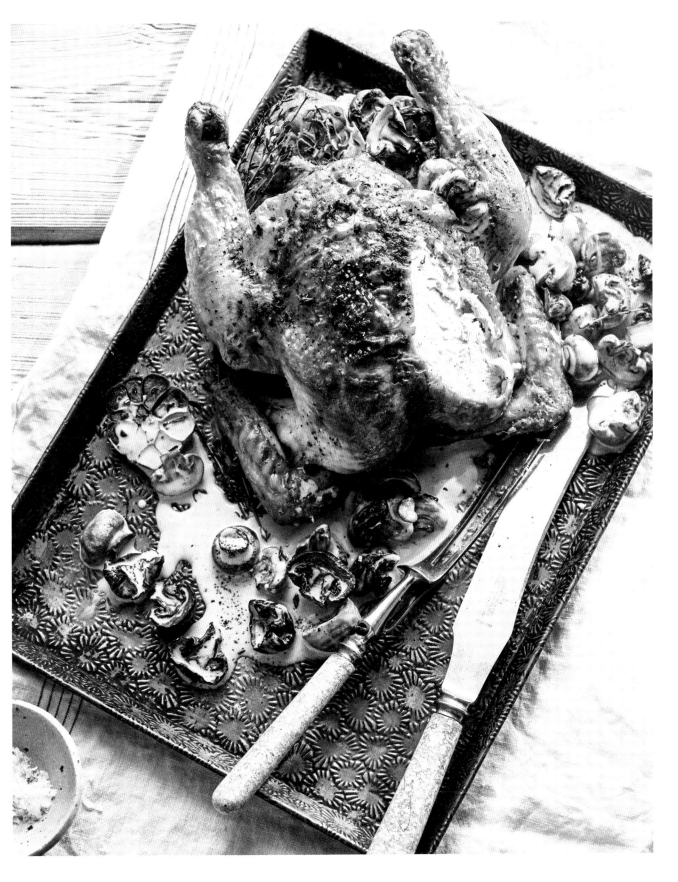

To make the mushroom and cream sauce, stir in the stock and crème fraîche. Taste and add seasoning as necessary. Transfer the sauce to a warm serving bowl and serve alongside the chicken.

To make the gravy, stir in the stock, add the butter and reduce for a few minutes over the heat. To thicken the gravy, make a runny paste from the arrowroot and a couple of tablespoons of water in a small bowl. Now whisk this into the gravy and bring it to a gentle boil. It will thicken as it heats. If you prefer a runnier gravy, add a little hot water; if you prefer it thicker, add a little more arrowroot paste. Taste and adjust the seasoning. Add a squeeze of lemon juice to taste, if you like. Serve with the chicken.

CHICKEN STOCK

U

MAKES APPROX. 3 LITRES (5¼ PINTS)

2–2.5kg (4lb 8oz–5lb 8oz) chicken
  carcasses and bones

4 litres (7 pints) cold water

1 medium white onion, unpeeled
  and roughly chopped, or a
  large handful of onion peelings

2 celery sticks with leaves,
  roughly chopped

1 leek top or 6 spring onion tops,
  roughly chopped (optional)

a small handful of flat-leaf parsley
  stalks (optional)

1 medium carrot, roughly chopped,
  or the same weight in peelings

6 black peppercorns

1 sprig of thyme

3 cloves

2 bay leaves

From one chicken you can make three meals: a simple, homely roast; a delicate and nourishing stock to use in a variety of other recipes; and soup and/or salads with the leftover meat. You will need more than one chicken carcass for this stock, but you can freeze one while you wait for another. I keep a bag of peelings from onions, leeks, carrots, celeriac and celery in the freezer and use them to make stock. Jenny loves to drink chicken stock with a pinch of salt during fasting hours, as it helps to break up the afternoon and also provides valuable electrolytes, especially sodium.

Put the chicken carcasses and any bones in a large saucepan, cover with the water and add the remaining ingredients. Bring to the boil, then reduce the heat to a gentle simmer. Cook for 3 hours, skimming the surface frequently to remove the foam, particularly at the beginning.

Strain the stock, reserving any large pieces of vegetables to eat cold or use in other recipes. Pick out any further flesh from the bones and set aside. Discard the remaining bones, giblets and cartilage. Use the stock straight away or store in the fridge for up to 4 days or freeze for up to 3 months. To save freezer space, it is a good idea to cook the strained stock for up to 1 hour longer to reduce it and concentrate the flavour.

Per serving
1.4g net carbs, 0g fibre,
8.3g protein, 4.6g fat, 81kcal

BONE BROTH

U
MAKES 1–2 LITRES (1¾–3½ PINTS)

2.5kg (5½lb) beef bones

2 carrots, roughly chopped, or the
    same weight in peelings

1 large white onion, cut into quarters

2 celery sticks, roughly chopped

a few celery leaves

a few flat-leaf parsley stalks

1 bay leaf

150ml (5fl oz) red wine

Per 100ml (3½fl oz) serving
3.7g net carbs, 0g fibre,
3.7g protein, 4.6g fat, 61kcal

This beefy broth is full of goodness and gentle flavour from the bones. It is ideal to drink when you are fasting and doesn't affect your glucose levels.

Preheat the oven to 220°C/200°C fan/425°F/gas mark 7. Put the bones, carrots, onion and celery into a roasting tin and roast for 1 hour. Halfway through, toss everything together. Remove from the oven and use tongs to transfer the bones and vegetables into your largest pot. Reserve the fat for future use.

Add the remaining ingredients and top up with cold water to cover the bones. Bring to the boil, then reduce the heat to a very gentle simmer. Cook for around 12 hours. Allow to cool before straining and storing.

LETTUCE CUPS WITH HAM, CHICKEN, TOMATOES & MAYO

SERVES 1

3 romaine lettuce leaves

150g (5½oz) cooked chicken or
    ham, cut into bite-sized pieces

6 cherry tomatoes, halved

1 celery stick, roughly chopped

a few celery, flat-leaf parsley,
    coriander or basil leaves,
    roughly chopped

2 tablespoons mayonnaise

a squeeze of lemon juice (optional)

salt and freshly ground black pepper

Per serving
5.3g net carbs, 3.7g fibre,
48.9g protein, 29.6g fat, 499kcal

This quick, light lunch is something we love to eat the day after a roast. Instead of bread, use long leaves of romaine lettuce as a vessel to hold meat, cheese, tomatoes, cooked fish or avocado. Then give it some flavour with herbs, lemon juice or hot sauce. I like to use celery for crunch but also for the leaves and their gentle spiciness.

Put the lettuce leaves in a wide bowl. Evenly divide the chicken, tomatoes, celery and herb leaves between them. Drop over the mayonnaise and squeeze over a little lemon juice, if using. Finish with a light scattering of salt and pepper. Enjoy.

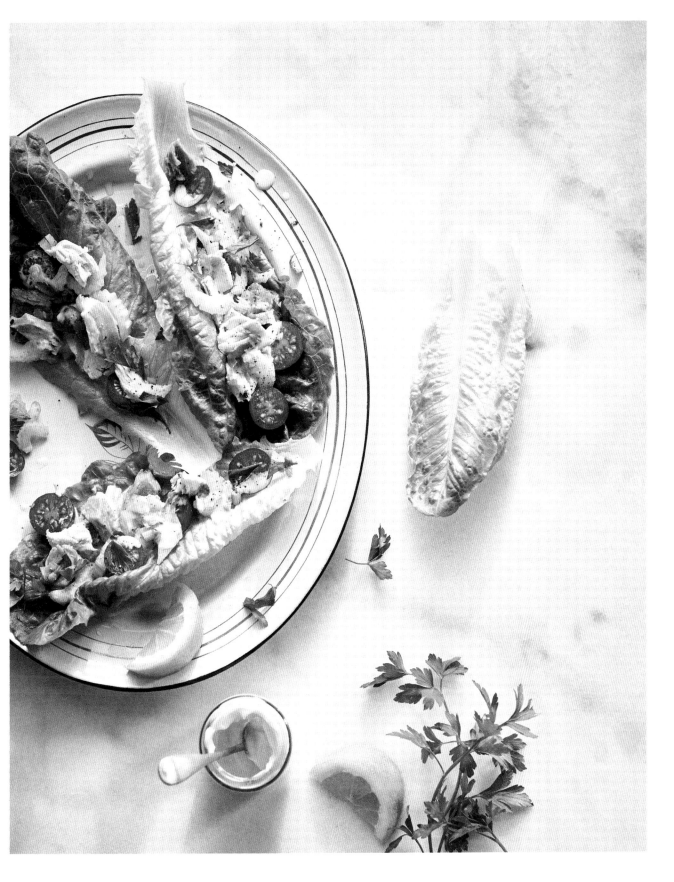

SPICY BUFFALO WINGS

MAKES 4

1kg (2lb 4oz) chicken wings
8 small gherkins (approx. 150g/5½oz),
    to serve

For the sauce
50g (1¾oz) chipotle or harissa paste
    or Frank's Original Red Hot sauce

Per serving of chicken
0.7g net carbs, 0.7g fibre,
60g protein, 42.5g fat, 641kcal

of slaw (optional)
5.7g net carbs, 2.2g fibre,
2.7g protein, 9.8g fat, 124kcal

I have always shied away from jars of paste and sauces, but as their quality has improved over the years, I now love the smoky heat of chipotle and harissa pastes as well as Frank's hot sauce, which is spicy and sugar-free. They all add flavour and spicy heat to chicken and all three are readily available both in supermarkets and online, so take your pick. The chicken wings are called "Buffalo" wings as the original recipe with Frank's hot sauce was created in Buffalo, NY. We love these with gherkins and either the Super slaw on page 166 or the Spicy avocado salad on page 162. This makes a substantial meal, so perhaps enjoy this on a day when you are enjoying other light meals.

Preheat the oven to 240°C/220°C fan/475°F/gas mark 9 or as hot as your oven will go.

Spread the chicken wings over a large ovenproof dish or roasting tray. Cook for 20–30 minutes or until golden brown, crispy and cooked through. They should be cooked after this time but to be sure, test the thickest part with a thermometer to check it is 80°C (176°F). If you don't have a meat thermometer, cut a thick wing open and make sure the meat isn't pink inside.

Meanwhile, stir the paste or sauce into 4 tablespoons of water in a large mixing bowl. Once the chicken is cooked, toss the wings into the bowl and thoroughly coat the wings in the sauce using 2 large spoons. Spread the wings back over the roasting tray and return it to the oven for 5 minutes. Remove from the oven and serve straight away with the gherkins and side of your choice.

GIANCARLO'S TUSCAN ROAST CHICKEN THIGHS

SERVES 4

4 tablespoons extra virgin olive oil

1 long sprig of rosemary

4 garlic cloves, skin on and
   lightly crushed

8 small chicken thighs, bone-in and
   skin on, approx. 1kg (2lb 4oz)

1 aubergine, cut into 3cm
   (1¼in) cubes

2 courgettes, cut into 3cm
   (1¼in) slices

8 cherry tomatoes

1 brown or red onion, cut into
   8 wedges

100ml (3½fl oz) dry white wine,
   stock or water

salt and freshly ground black pepper

Per serving
7.6g net carbs, 5.7g fibre,
67g protein, 37g fat, 648kcal

This is an all-in-one, easy, versatile recipe that can be left in the oven to cook while you get on with something else. It doesn't have to be made with chicken thighs – a jointed chicken also works well, although bigger pieces might need longer to cook. Alter the vegetables according to what you have in the fridge – cubes of pumpkin, swede or butternut squash add colour and natural sweetness. Italians cook chicken such as this for a long time so that the meat falls from the bones and the skin crispens to a rich golden brown.

Preheat the oven to 180°C/160°C fan/350°F/gas mark 4.

Drizzle a little of the oil over a roasting tray and lay the rosemary and garlic on the base. Season the chicken thighs all over with salt and pepper and put them on top, skin-side up. Arrange the vegetables around the chicken and season. Pour the rest of the oil over the chicken and vegetables and roast for 30 minutes.

Remove the tray from the oven and baste the chicken and vegetables with the cooking juices. Pour the white wine around the chicken but not over the crispy skin.

Return the chicken to the oven and roast for a further 20–30 minutes or until cooked through and the meat falls from the bones (the cooking time will depend on the size of the thighs). Serve with the juices from the pan poured over the chicken.

CHICKEN SOUVLAKI

L

SERVES 4

For the marinade

1 teaspoon ground coriander

1 teaspoon dried oregano

1 teaspoon sweet paprika

1 fat garlic clove, grated

1 teaspoon ground black pepper

2 teaspoons lemon juice

1 teaspoon hot sauce (optional)

1 tablespoon dark soy sauce

3 tablespoons extra virgin olive oil

For the skewers

2 skinless chicken breasts or boneless, skinless thighs, approx. 400g (14oz), cut into 3cm (1¼in) cubes

1 small onion, cut into 3cm (1¼in) wedges and petals separated

1 red pepper, cut into 3cm (1¼in) squares

lemon wedges, to serve (optional)

Per serving

2.9g net carbs, 0.9g fibre, 31.4g protein, 14.8g fat, 278kcal

Whether we use the grill indoors in winter or the barbecue in summer, our family loves kebabs. I like the fact I can make them in advance and quickly thread them on to skewers while the grill heats up. They cook in less than 15 minutes and look and taste amazing. These souvlaki work well with any of the salads from the Sides chapter or the Cucumber & tomato raita on page 181.

The souvlaki and the following kebab recipe require a marinade to be applied to the chicken before cooking. This marinade is via our friend Brian McLeod, who was inspired by years of living in Cyprus. For a marinade to work you need an acid (in the form of yogurt or lemon juice in this case), oil and flavourings. Both require at least 30 minutes to work but can be left overnight in the fridge.

Thoroughly mix all the marinade ingredients together in a non-metallic bowl.

Add the chicken, onion petals and red pepper to the bowl and mix again to coat all the ingredients. Cover and refrigerate for a minimum of 30 minutes or overnight.

Meanwhile, soak any wooden skewers, if using, in water and line a grill tray or baking tray with foil. Heat the grill to hot or fire up the barbecue.

Thread the chicken and vegetables alternately on to your skewers. Cook them close to the hot grill for 5–7 minutes until they are just browned. Turn the kebabs and grill again for 5 minutes until cooked through. The timing will depend on how close the rack is to the heat source.

To make sure the chicken is cooked through, cut the fattest piece in half to make sure there are no pink juices inside. Alternatively, use a thermometer to measure the thickest piece; it should be 80°C (176°F). Serve the skewers as soon as they are cooked with a salad of your choice and lemon wedges, if you wish.

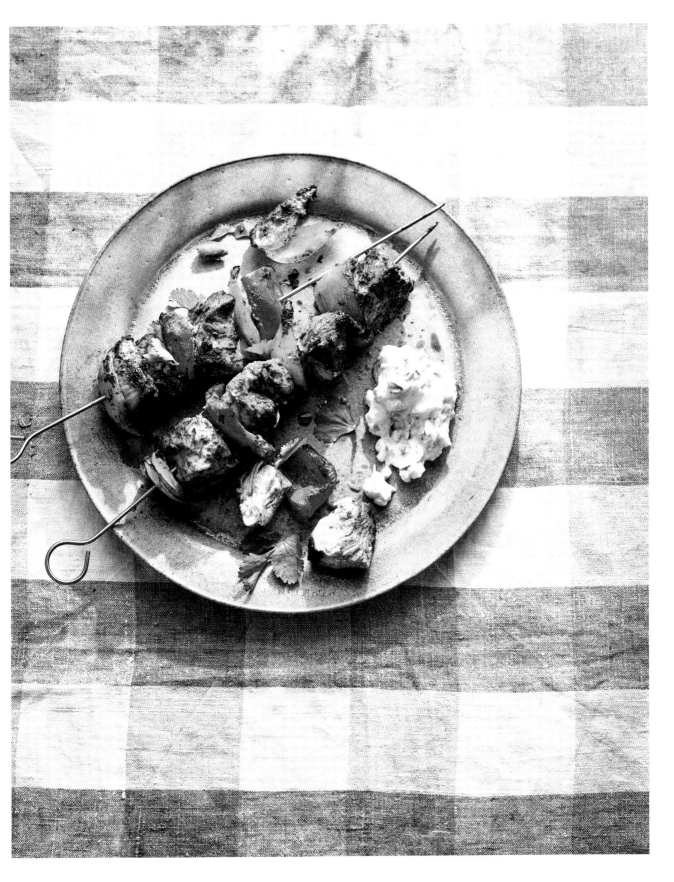

SPICED CORIANDER CHICKEN KEBABS

L

SERVES 4

For the marinade

25g (1oz) coriander

2 fat garlic cloves

a thumb-sized piece of fresh ginger

1 hot small green chilli

2 tablespoons olive oil or ghee

1 tablespoon lemon juice

1 tablespoon chicken tikka powder

1 teaspoon salt

75g (2¾oz) Greek yogurt

For the skewers

2 skinless chicken breasts or
 boneless, skinless thighs,
 approx. 400g (14oz), cut into
 3cm (1¼in) cubes

1 small onion, cut into 3cm (1¼in)
 wedges and petals separated

1 red pepper, cut into 3cm
 (1¼in) squares

lemon wedges, to serve (optional)

Per serving
4.5g net carbs, 1.1g fibre,
32.8g protein, 12.9g fat, 274kcal

This marinade was inspired by a trip to Kolkata. I suggest you serve the kebabs with salads or with the Vibrant vegetable korma on pages 156–157 and/or the Cucumber & tomato raita on page 181.

Blend the coriander, garlic, ginger and chilli with the olive oil and lemon juice in a food processor. Transfer to a non-metallic bowl and stir in the chicken tikka powder, salt and yogurt. Alternatively, cut the coriander and chilli finely by hand and grate the garlic and ginger, then mix together with the remaining ingredients.

Add the chicken, onion petals and red pepper to the bowl and mix again to coat all the ingredients. Cover and refrigerate for a minimum of 30 minutes or overnight.

Meanwhile, soak any wooden skewers, if using, in water and line a grill tray or baking tray with foil. Heat the grill to hot or fire up the barbecue.

Thread the chicken and vegetables alternately on to your skewers. Cook them close to the hot grill for 5–7 minutes until they are just browned. Turn the kebabs and grill again for 5 minutes until cooked through. The timing will depend on how close the rack is to the heat source.

To make sure the chicken is cooked through, cut the fattest piece in half to make sure there are no pink juices inside. Alternatively, use a thermometer to measure the thickest piece; it should be 80°C (176°F). Serve the skewers as soon as they are cooked with a side of your choice and lemon wedges, if you wish.

ONE-POT SAUSAGE, PEPPER & TOMATO STEW

SERVES 4

3 tablespoons extra virgin olive oil

1 onion, finely sliced into half-moons

1 green or yellow pepper, roughly
  cubed into bite-sized pieces

200g (7oz) mushrooms, halved or
  quartered if large (optional)

400g (14oz) high-meat-content
  pork or beef sausages or
  lean diced pork

1 fat garlic clove, finely sliced
  or crushed

a few sprigs of thyme or 1 teaspoon
  dried thyme

1–2 teaspoons sweet, hot or smoked
  paprika, or a pinch of each

400g (14oz) fresh or can of
  chopped tomatoes

400g (14oz) can of chickpeas,
  drained

approx. 100g (3½oz) spinach, chard
  or beet leaves

salt and freshly ground black pepper

Per serving
17g net carbs, 4.8g fibre,
27g protein, 33g fat, 483kcal

This lazy one-pot dish is loosely based on *katino meze*, a Bulgarian appetizer which we loved on our trip to the wonderful cities of Sofia and Plovdiv. It is usually made with pork, but I find chopped sausages even easier to use and they add more flavour. To keep the carbs down, look for high-meat-content sausages rather than those filled with rusk or flour. I add green leaves to the dish to make it a whole meal, which I serve in bowls.

If I am making this for the family, I take some out for Giancarlo and then add the can of drained chickpeas or beans for the boys to make it more filling. It is a great way to use up soft tomatoes too. The paprika can be sweet (mild), hot, smoked or unsmoked – in fact I like mainly sweet with a pinch of hot for flavour and heat. Serve it as it is or add grated cheese or soured cream.

Heat the oil in a large frying pan or wok over a medium–high heat. Add the onion and a little seasoning and cook for about 5 minutes before adding the pepper and mushrooms, if using. Stir occasionally.

Meanwhile, cut the sausages into bite-sized pieces; depending on the strength of the skins you can do this with scissors straight into the pan or sometimes it's easier to squeeze the sausage meat out of the skins and drop it into the pan. Add the garlic and stir through, then cook for 7–10 minutes, stirring frequently, until the sausages are browned on all sides. Stir in the thyme and 1 teaspoon of the paprika.

Coarsely grate the fresh tomatoes, if using, on to a plate and discard the skins. Add these or the canned tomatoes and drained chickpeas. Stir again and bring to the boil. Cook for a few minutes until the sausages are cooked through. Taste and add seasoning and paprika as necessary. Stir in your choice of leaves and pop the lid back on. As soon as the leaves have wilted – spinach will take about 3 minutes and kale will take up to 10 minutes – the stew is ready to serve.

SLOW-COOKED PULLED PORK

SERVES 6

1.2–1.4kg (2lb 11oz–3lb 3oz) boneless or bone-in pork shoulder, string removed, or meaty pork ribs

1 teaspoon salt and plenty of freshly ground black pepper

3 tablespoons extra virgin olive oil

1 medium onion, finely chopped

4 fat garlic cloves, peeled and lightly squashed

¼ teaspoon chilli flakes

2 teaspoons ground cumin

1 teaspoon smoked chipotle powder or smoked hot paprika

1 teaspoon fresh or dried thyme or oregano

3 tablespoons cider or wine vinegar

1 tablespoon Worcestershire sauce

3 tablespoons tomato purée

Per serving
5.3g net carbs, 1.7g fibre, 68g protein, 25g fat, 531kcal

This classic American recipe is something we have all grown to love over recent years. It's often loaded with sugar, but you can easily make your own sugar-free version in the oven or a slow cooker. If the casserole can be used on the hob or the slow cooker has a sauté option, then all the better as this will be a one-pot dish. This is a hot and spicy sauce, if you prefer it mild, use regular sweet paprika and omit the chilli. If you don't want to use pork shoulder, economical meaty ribs work just as well. We serve this with the Super slaw on page 162, Avocado mash (page 149) and gherkins.

If you have a slow cooker that browns, then do use this for the first part of the recipe. If it doesn't or your casserole doesn't work with your hob, then make the first part of the recipe in a large frying pan.

Preheat the oven to 190°C/170°C fan/375°F/gas mark 5 or your slow cooker to sauté.

Season the pork and brown all over in the oil – this will take about 7–10 minutes. Add the onion and garlic to the pan and let these soften for 5 minutes, stirring frequently around the pork. Now add the spices and stir to combine with the onion. Add the remaining ingredients and 400ml (14fl oz) water to the casserole or slow cooker and bring to the boil. Put on the lid.

If using a casserole, cook the pork shoulder in the oven for 3 hours and the ribs for 1½–2 hours or until the meat falls apart easily. Turn the shoulder or the ribs halfway through cooking and top up with a little hot water if it looks dry.

If using a slow cooker, cook on low for 6–8 hours for the shoulder, depending on the size, and about 5 hours for ribs, turning halfway through cooking until the pork falls apart easily. Top up with a little hot water if it looks dry.

When the pork is done, transfer it to a chopping board. Use 2 forks to pull the meat apart into shreds. Depending on your cut of pork there may be a lot of fat on the surface of the sauce. Use a spoon to collect most of it and discard. Return the pulled pork shoulder to the sauce and heat through. Serve warm. You can do the same with the ribs or serve them as they are with the sauce on the side, which can be left as it is or puréed smooth.

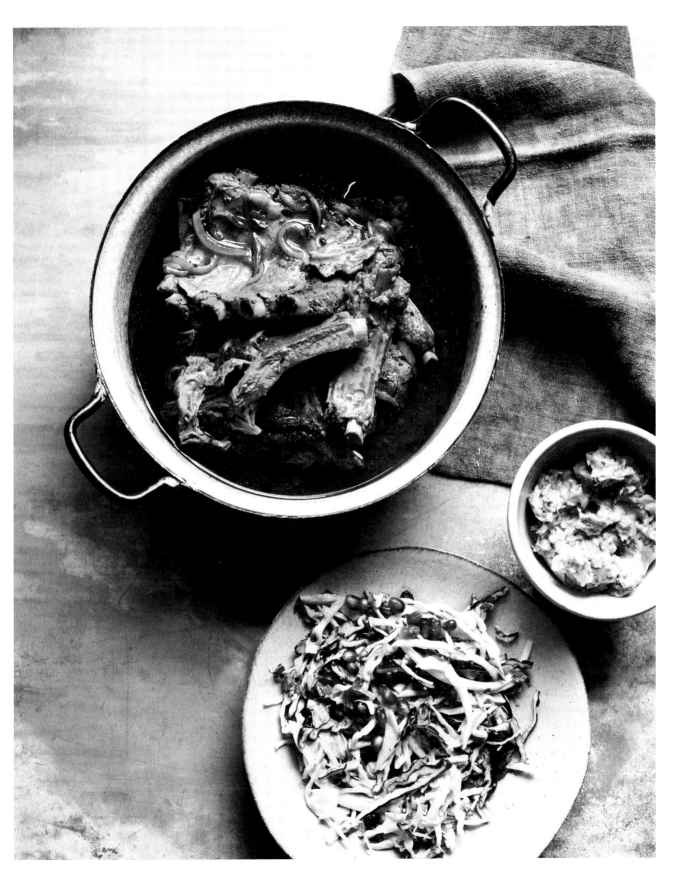

MIGHTY MEATLOAF

L

SERVES 6

8 thin rashers (approx. 125g/4½oz) smoked streaky bacon

50g (1¾oz) oats

1 medium onion

1 courgette

30g (1oz) mature Cheddar or Parmesan cheese, grated

500g (1lb 2oz) pork or beef mince or a mixture of the two

2 teaspoons fresh or dried finely chopped sage, thyme or rosemary

2 eggs

1 teaspoon salt and plenty of freshly ground black pepper

Per serving
7.2g net carbs, 1.5g fibre, 25.2g protein, 12.7g fat, 250kcal

This is a hybrid of Jenny's meatloaf recipe and mine. We both love to make meatloaf as it is simple, inexpensive and gives you leftovers to enjoy the following day. Swap out the pork for beef or lamb mince, but if you miss out the bacon rashers, then line the tin with a piece of baking parchment.

Lay the bacon rashers, slightly overlapping, so that they cover the long sides and base of a 900g (2lb) loaf tin – don't worry about the short ends.

Preheat the oven to 200°C/180°C fan/400°F/gas mark 6.

If the oats are coarse, jumbo style, pulse them in a food processor to a finer texture; they don't have to be a powder but just chopped finely to help absorb the juices. Do this by hand if you don't have a food processor. Tip into a mixing bowl. Now use the food processor to chop the onion and courgette finely, or coarsely grate them by hand. Add these to the bowl with the remaining ingredients and mix thoroughly with your hands.

Pack the mixture into the bacon-lined tin, being careful not to dislodge the rashers. If any rashers are still visible, fold them over the top of the mixture to encase it.

Bake the meatloaf for 45 minutes or until firm to the touch and cooked through. Remove the loaf from the oven and increase the oven temperature to 220°C/200°C fan/425°F/gas mark 7. Invert the meatloaf tin on to a roasting tray. Wipe away any juices that have leaked out of the meat and return the meatloaf to the oven for 7–10 minutes to crispen and brown the bacon. Transfer to a serving dish and eat straight away or keep it warm for up to 30 minutes before serving.

BOEUF BOURGUIGNON

SERVES 8

5 tablespoons extra virgin olive oil

50g (1¾oz) butter

1.5kg (3lb 5oz) stewing beef, cut into bite-sized pieces

1 large onion, roughly chopped

200g (7oz) pancetta, cubed, or unsmoked bacon lardons

1 celery stick, roughly chopped

1 large carrot, roughly chopped

5 fat garlic cloves, peeled and lightly squashed

a few sprigs of thyme, plus extra to serve

2 bay leaves

500ml (18fl oz) red wine

500ml (18fl oz) beef stock

1 large leek, washed and cut into 2cm (¾in) slices

250g (9oz) small whole button mushrooms, or chestnut mushrooms, halved

2 tablespoons cornflour (optional)

salt and freshly ground black pepper

Per serving without cornflour
7.6g net carbs, 1.9g fibre,
63g protein, 21g fat, 473kcal

If you have never made this classic French stew, make a vow to give it a go – it won't disappoint. Good cuts of beef for this are the cheaper ones that have enough collagen to produce soft, tender meat that doesn't dry out during the long, slow cook; cheek, fatty brisket and chuck are perfect for the task.

I have swapped pieces of leek for the button onions to give more colour and natural sweetness and to reduce the carbs and the work. This is lovely with soft, buttered ribbons of any cabbage, a green seasonal vegetable or vegetable mash (see page 173). It is ideal to reheat, freezes well and can be taken to work to reheat in the microwave; great for making your work colleagues jealous as they eat their soggy sandwiches.

Heat 3 tablespoons of the oil and half the butter in a large, heavy-based casserole or saucepan (with a lid). Sear one third of the beef until it is a rich, dark brown all over. Using a slotted spoon, transfer the meat to a warm bowl. Repeat with the other two thirds of the beef. Keep the oil and juices in the pan and fry the onion, pancetta, celery, carrot and garlic with the herbs, 2 teaspoons of salt and some black pepper for 12–15 minutes until soft.

Now, return the meat to the casserole and stir through. Pour in the wine and stock and stir. Bring to the boil, then reduce the heat and cook very gently so that the surface is just trembling, uncovered, for 2 hours. If it starts to look dry, add a splash of hot water and put the lid on.

Meanwhile, fry the leek and mushrooms in the remaining olive oil and butter with seasoning for about 15 minutes or until lightly browned. After 2 hours, add the leeks and mushrooms to the casserole and gently stir through. Continue to cook for 30 minutes–1 hour. Taste the sauce and adjust the seasoning accordingly. Remove the casserole from the heat and leave to settle off the heat for a couple of minutes and skim off any excess fat. If the sauce is very watery, it can be thickened with the addition of the cornflour mixed with 2 tablespoons of water. Stir and heat until thickened.

Serve in warm bowls with sprigs of thyme and buttery celeriac mash.

THE MAGNIFICENT MIXED GRILL

SERVES 2

2 large portobello mushrooms (approx. 220g/8oz)

2 tablespoons extra virgin olive oil

2 high-meat-content sausages

2 medium tomatoes, halved

½ teaspoon dried oregano

1 sirloin or rib-eye steak, approx. 200g (7oz), with a fat edge

a handful of watercress, rocket or lamb's lettuce

For the garlic butter

15g (½oz) butter, softened

1 small garlic clove, crushed or grated

1 heaped teaspoon finely chopped celery leaves, chives or flat-leaf parsley

salt and freshly ground black pepper

Per serving
6.1g net carbs, 3.1g fibre, 41g protein, 30g fat, 466kcal

When I was growing up in Eastbourne my birthday treat was to go to our local Italian restaurant; my favourite meal was a mixed grill. I remember the waiters making a fuss of me – this little girl with this huge plate of food! I loved the variety of meats, grilled tomatoes and garlic mushrooms. Little did I know I would marry an Italian and we would have two restaurants. I also didn't know then that I was choosing to eat a perfect low-carb dish!

Choose high-meat-content sausages that contain little or no rusk or tapioca starch to keep the carbs low and use the remainder in the One-pot sausage, pepper & tomato stew on page 115.

Preheat the grill to hot. Let the steak come to room temperature.

To make the garlic butter, remove the stalks from the mushrooms and finely chop them. Transfer to a small bowl and mix them with the garlic butter ingredients, ¼ teaspoon of salt and plenty of black pepper. Set aside.

Put the stalkless mushrooms, domed-side up, on a grill rack over an oven tray to catch the juices. Brush over a little of the olive oil. Put the sausages next to them and grill, close to the heat source, for 5 minutes.

Cut the tomatoes in half around the middle (they are prettier cut this way) and drizzle with a little of the remaining olive oil. Scatter over the oregano and season with salt and pepper. Set aside.

Remove the rack and tray. Turn the sausages and mushrooms. Spread the garlic butter over the gill side of the mushrooms using a knife. Add the tomatoes to the rack and grill for 5–10 minutes or until the sausages are cooked, the mushrooms are lightly browned and wrinkled around the edges and the tomatoes have softened. Keep an eye on the grill as the cooking times will depend on the heat of your grill and how close the rack is to the heat. Turn the sausages as necessary.

Meanwhile, heat a small frying pan over a high heat. Season the steak generously all over. Hold the steak fat-side down in the hot frying pan with tongs. Let it sizzle, brown and release the fat, then use that to cook the steak. A 2cm (¾in) thick sirloin or rib-eye steak will take about 1½ minutes a side for rare, 2 minutes a side for medium rare and 3 minutes a side for medium. Remove from the pan and set aside in a warm place to rest.

When everything is cooked, divide between 2 warm plates. Pour over any cooking juices from the tray. Serve with watercress.

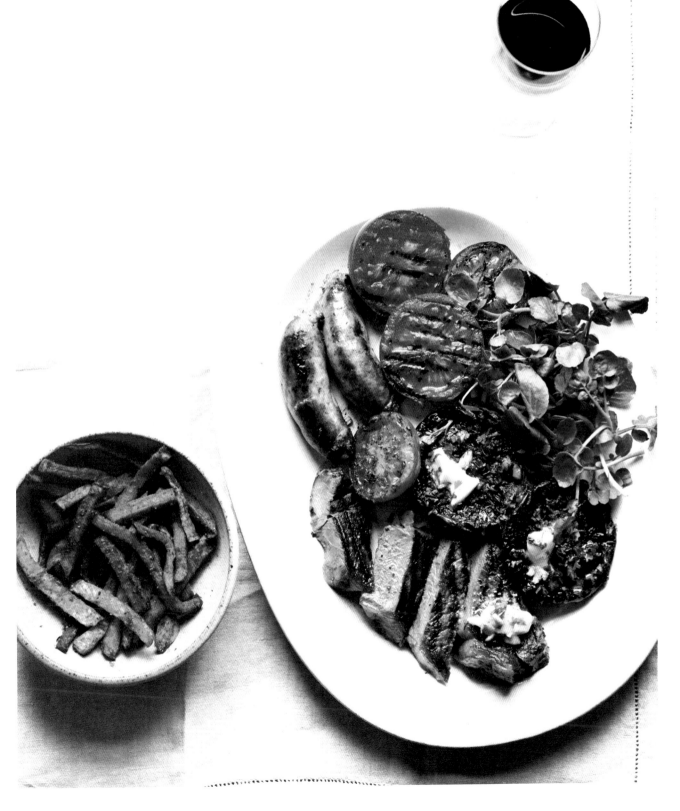

SLOW-COOKED LAMB CURRY

L   lamb curry

G   lamb curry with pilao cauli rice

SERVES 8

2 medium onions, finely chopped

½ teaspoon ground cloves or
    4 cloves

1 cinnamon stick

2 tablespoons ghee

2 tablespoons coriander seeds

2 tablespoons cumin seeds

1 star anise

400g (14oz) can of chopped
    tomatoes

4 fat garlic cloves, grated

10g (¼oz) fresh ginger, peeled
    and grated

2 small, hot red chillies,
    finely chopped

1 heaped teaspoon salt

1 medium aubergine

1.2kg (2lb 11oz) stewing lamb,
    cut into 3cm (1¼in) dice

a large handful (10g/¼oz) of
    coriander, roughly chopped,
    plus extra to serve

1 tablespoon tomato purée

½ teaspoon garam masala (optional)

Per serving
6.8g net carbs, 2.5g fibre,
42g protein, 22g fat, 396kcal

with pilao cauli rice
13.6g net carbs, 5.9g fibre,
45.2g protein, 32g fat, 534kcal

This recipe is from our friend Preeti Gohil. It is her family's way of making curry; they are from Kenya, but Preeti thinks the recipe is originally from Gujarat in Western India. She makes a ground spice mix called *dhana jeera* from roasted coriander and cumin and a star anise. Preeti's family use grated aubergine to give a wonderful creamy consistency to the curry.

The base sauce of the curry is very versatile; since Preeti is vegetarian but her family eat meat, she takes some of the cooked sauce out of the pan before adding the meat. When the family are ready to eat, she cracks two eggs into the sauce in a small pan, puts a lid on and cooks the eggs, then serves them scattered with garam masala and coriander. Preeti told me you can also use beef in place of the lamb or swap in chicken thighs, in which case she leaves the aubergine out.

Cook the onions, cloves and cinnamon in the ghee in a heavy-based casserole with a lid for 30 minutes or until very soft and brown. Keep the lid on and stir every now and again.

Meanwhile, make the *dhana jeera* spice mix by dry-frying the coriander and cumin seeds with the star anise in a small frying pan for about 2 minutes or until they turn a shade darker and smell amazing. Tip them on to a piece of baking parchment to cool, then fold the parchment and shoot them into a spice grinder, small food processor or pestle and mortar. Grind to a fine powder.

Add the tomatoes to the onions, followed by the garlic, ginger, chillies, salt and *dhana jeera*. Peel the aubergine and coarsely grate into the casserole. Stir through and cook for 10 minutes until the aubergine has softened.

Add the lamb and fresh coriander and stir through. Bring to the boil, then reduce the heat to low and cook, covered, for 1½ hours or until the lamb is tender and flakes easily. Alternatively, cook the curry in a slow cooker for about 5 hours; although if you wanted to leave it for up to 8 hours or overnight, it will also be fine.

Ten minutes before serving, stir in the tomato purée and continue to cook. Just before serving, scatter over the garam masala, if using, and some coriander. Serve the curry with the Pilao cauli rice on page 93 and/or the Chapattis on page 92.

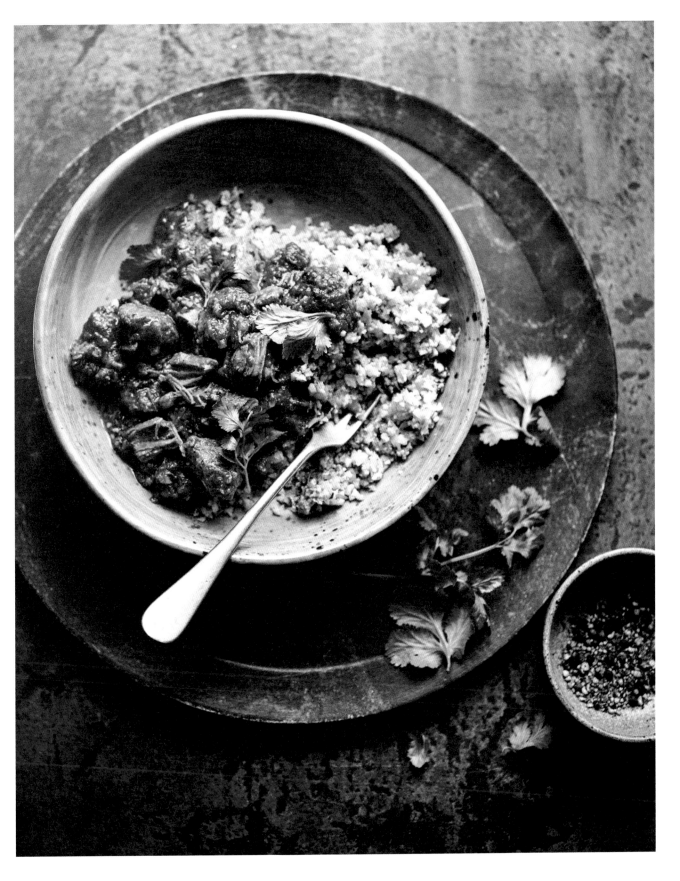

SWEDISH MEATBALLS IN CREAM SAUCE WITH BERRY JAM

SERVES 6

4 tablespoons ghee, olive oil or beef dripping

3 tablespoons finely chopped dill or chives

salt and freshly ground black pepper

For the meatballs

500g (1lb 2oz) 15% fat minced beef

250g (9oz) 15–20% fat pork mince

1 onion, finely chopped

2 fat garlic cloves, finely chopped or grated

1 egg

25g (1oz) flat-leaf parsley, leaves and stems finely chopped

1 teaspoon dried or fresh thyme leaves, plus extra to serve

1 teaspoon grated nutmeg

1 teaspoon ground allspice

For the cream sauce

400ml (14fl oz) beef stock

200ml (7fl oz) double cream

2 tablespoons Worcestershire sauce

2 teaspoons Dijon mustard

For the berry jam

300g (10½oz) frozen or fresh mixed berries, such as raspberries, blackberries, strawberries and redcurrants

1 tablespoon erythritol or 2 teaspoons honey

It was the furniture shop IKEA that brought Swedish meatballs to the rest of the world, and we all fell in love with the mildly spiced patties served in a creamy sauce. I like them with the Sautéed greens on page 167 or the Brussels sprout, bacon & leek hash on page 176.

Put all the meatball ingredients into a mixing bowl with 1 teaspoon of salt and plenty of black pepper and use your hands to thoroughly mix together. Make up a small patty about the size of your thumb tip and flatten gently. Fry this on both sides in a little oil in a large non-stick frying pan. Remove from the pan when cooked through and taste it. Now alter the seasoning as necessary for the rest of the batch.

When you are happy with the seasoning, make up the rest of the meatballs by rolling the mixture into walnut-sized balls. You should have about 45 of these. Fry these in batches in the ghee until browned on all sides and cooked through.

To make the cream sauce, put all the ingredients into a saucepan. Bring to the boil and then reduce the heat to a simmer. Let it bubble slowly for 5–10 minutes to reduce to a thick, coating consistency. Taste and add salt gingerly, as some stocks are already salty.

To make the jam, mash the berries with a potato masher in a saucepan over a medium heat. You can do this from frozen, there is no need to defrost them. Once they release their juices, add the erythritol or honey and mash again to mix. Transfer the jam to a serving bowl.

To serve, put the meatballs into a warm serving dish, pour over the cream sauce and scatter over the dill or chives. Serve with the jam alongside.

Per serving of meatballs in the sauce
2.9g net carbs, 0.4g fibre, 27.4g protein, 43.3g fat, 510kcal

of jam with honey
5.2g net carbs, 3.4g fibre, 0.6g protein, 0.2g fat, 31kcal

of jam with erythritol
3.3g net carbs, 3.4g fibre, 0.6g protein, 0.2g fat, 24kcal

QUICK & SPICY STIR-FRIED LAMB MINCE

L

SERVES 4

2 tablespoons ghee or extra
    virgin olive oil

1 onion, sliced into half-moons

2 fat garlic cloves, crushed

500g (1lb 2oz) minced lamb

1 teaspoon ground cumin

pinch of chilli flakes (optional)

1 teaspoon dried oregano

2 tablespoons tomato purée

salt and plenty of ground
    black pepper

**For the lamb mince with
cheesy topping**

3 eggs

75g (2¾oz) Cheddar or feta
    cheese, coarsely grated

For the wraps

6 coconut and coriander crêpes
    (page 79)

250g (9oz) Greek yogurt

a small handful of coriander leaves,
    to serve (optional)

I love to make this quick dish and use it in a variety of ways. The mince is lovely served in bowls with Cauli rice (page 93), or it makes the perfect stuffing for the Coconut crêpes on page 79, or you can add a cheesy topping and serve it straight from the pan. I have also used this mince to add extra protein to the Aubergine parmigiana on page 147; it's wonderful and almost makes it into a moussaka.

Heat the ghee or oil in a large frying pan or wok and fry the onion over a medium–high heat for about 10 minutes until it starts to brown and soften. Add the garlic, minced lamb, seasoning, spices and herbs and stir through. Keep bashing the meat with a wooden spoon to break up any lumps. Continue to cook for 10–15 minutes until the meat is lightly browned and cooked through and any water has evaporated.

Mix the tomato purée with 75ml (2½fl oz) water in a mug and add to the pan. Cook for 5 minutes, then taste and adjust the seasoning to your liking. Serve straight away or keep warm until you are ready.

For the lamb mince with cheesy topping, beat the eggs with the cheese in a bowl and, when the lamb is just cooked, pour this into the pan. Put a lid on the pan and continue to cook over a low heat for 7–10 minutes or until the egg is set and cooked. Serve straight away.

For the wraps, spread each wrap with a couple of teaspoons of yogurt towards one side. Divide the lamb between them, add a few leaves of coriander and roll up.

Per serving
of mince
4.1g net carbs, 1.2g fibre, 26g protein, 16g fat, 271kcal

with cheese topping
4.6g net carbs, 1.2g fibre, 36g protein, 27g fat, 406kcal

Per filled wrap
11g net carbs, 2.7g fibre, 23g protein, 13g fat, 267kcal

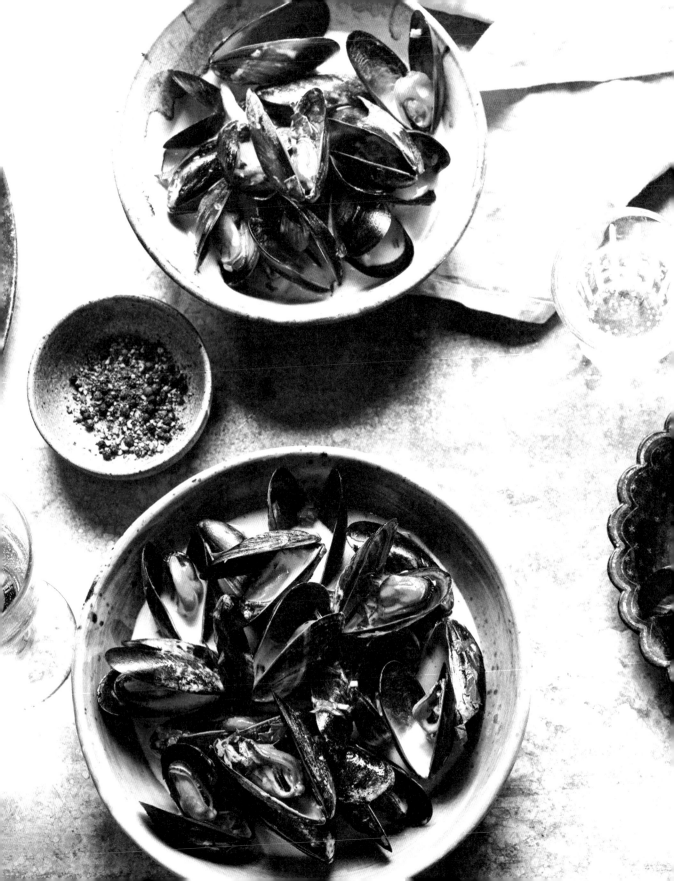

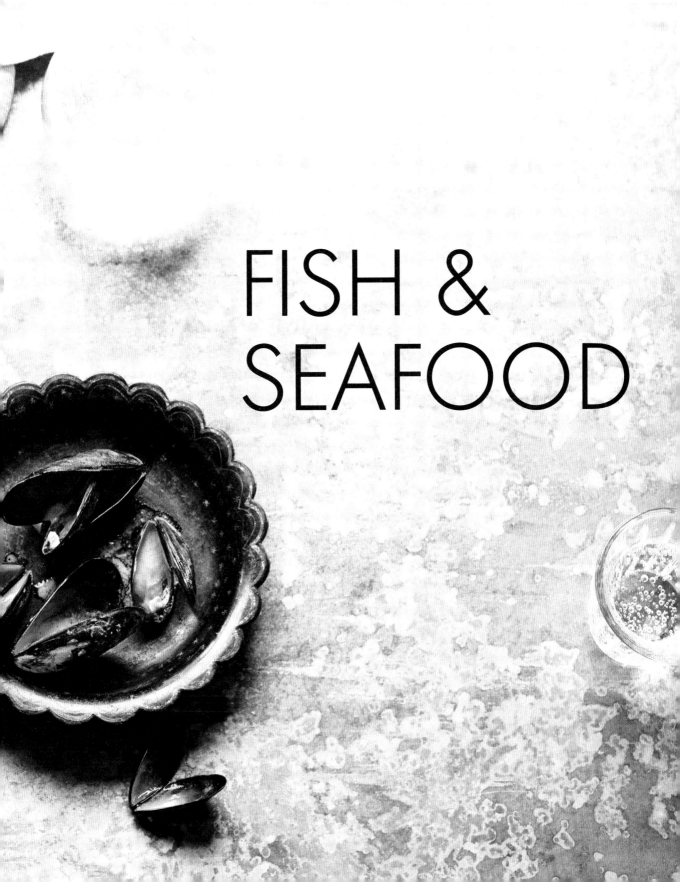

FISH &
SEAFOOD

SMOKED SALMON SALAD

L

SERVES 2

½ small red onion, finely chopped

125g (4½oz) romaine or little
   gem lettuce or watercress

120g (4¼oz) smoked or hot-smoked
   salmon

4 soft-boiled eggs, peeled

1 tablespoon capers, rinsed and
   roughly chopped if large

salt and freshly ground black pepper

For the dressing

2 tablespoons Greek yogurt

2 tablespoons mayonnaise

2 teaspoons lemon juice

finely grated zest of ½ lemon

Per serving
4.5g net carbs, 1.8g fibre,
23.7g protein, 27.6g fat, 369kcal

This oh-so-simple salad can be whipped up in minutes but never ceases to impress. It has all the right components: crunchy lettuce, soft eggs and salmon, punchy capers and a creamy dressing. It's perfect for a light brunch or lunch and is surprisingly filling; however, if you're after something even more substantial, then add a slice of the Country-style loaf on page 64. Use any salad leaves you have in, ideally something crunchy, such as romaine, and another leaf with bite, such as watercress or rocket.

Soak the onion in a bowl of cold water.

Trim the lettuce of any tough stems, roughly chop and separate any tightly packed lettuce leaves; scatter them between 2 plates. Tear the salmon into bite-sized pieces and divide these between the 2 plates. Cut the eggs in half and add these and the capers.

Mix together the dressing ingredients, taste and adjust the seasoning as necessary. Spoon this over the salad. Drain the onion and scatter over. Season with a little salt over the eggs and plenty of black pepper. Serve straight away.

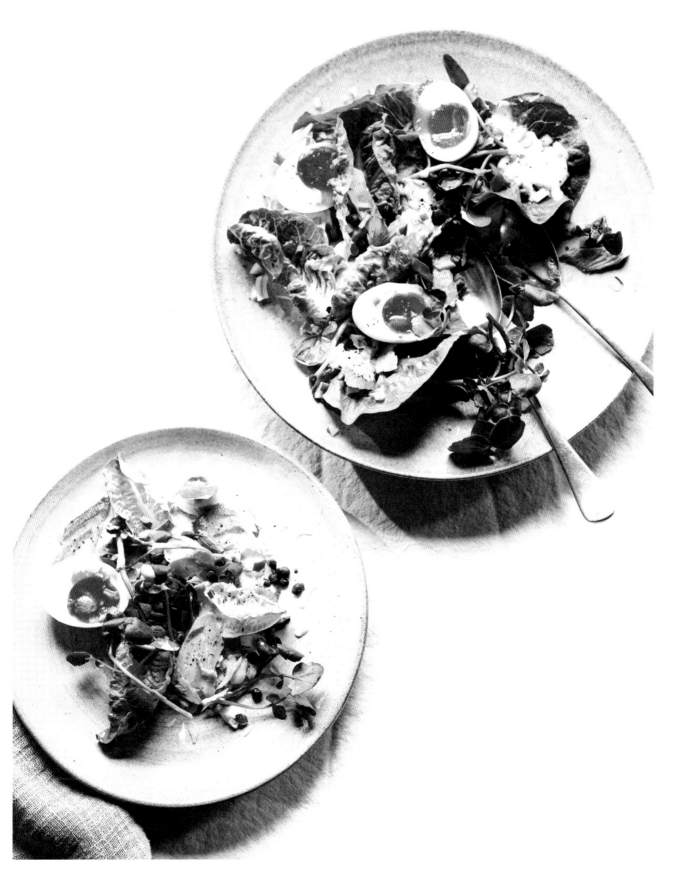

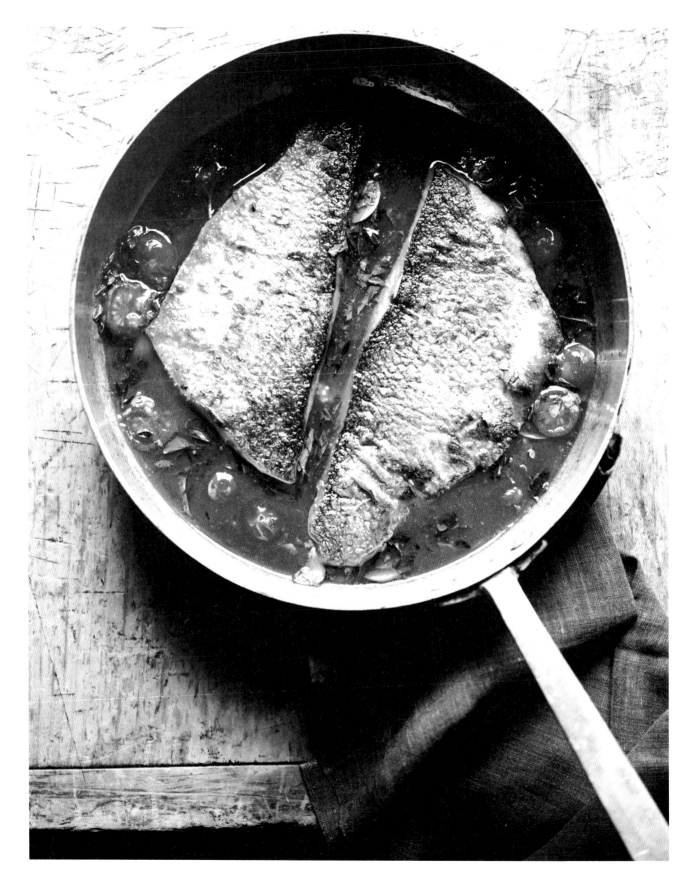

SEA BASS IN ACQUA PAZZA

G with a side of your choice
SERVES 2

4 tablespoons extra virgin olive oil

2 sea bass or bream fillets, skin on

1 fat garlic clove, finely sliced

½ red chilli, depending on strength, finely chopped

10 cherry tomatoes, halved

1 teaspoon tomato purée

75ml (2½fl oz) dry white wine

75ml (2½fl oz) just-boiled water

1 sprig of thyme or ½ teaspoon dried thyme (optional)

a handful of flat-leaf parsley, roughly chopped

salt and freshly ground black pepper

Per serving
6.2g net carbs, 2.2g fibre,
19g protein, 34g fat, 447kcal

Gregorio Piazza, our Head Chef at Caldesi in Campagna, showed me how to cook this dish. It's all about cooking fish quickly in water (*acqua*) that is turned "crazy" (*pazza*) with the addition of tomatoes, chilli and salt. This is best done with the ripest, most flavourful tomatoes you can lay your hands on. Do taste your chilli to know how hot it is, so that you know how much to add. Serve this with green beans, broccoli or spinach.

Heat half the oil in a large frying pan over a medium heat. Season the fish all over with salt and a little pepper. Fry the fish fillets for about 5 minutes, skin-side down, until the skin is crisp. Transfer the fish to a warm plate and set aside; discard the oil from the pan.

Add the remaining 2 tablespoons of oil to the pan and fry the garlic, chilli and cherry tomatoes for a minute, making sure that the garlic doesn't burn. Add the tomato purée, wine, just-boiled water, thyme and parsley and bring to the boil. Allow it to boil like crazy until the liquor reduces by half – this should take about 5 minutes. Return the fish to the pan, skin-side up, and cook in the sauce for just 2 minutes.

Serve the fish with the sauce on warm plates, with your choice of vegetables.

TUNA, AVOCADO & MANGO CEVICHE

L

SERVES 4

3 spring onions or ½ small red onion,
  finely chopped

250g (9oz) raw sushi-grade tuna or
  salmon, or cooked prawns

150g (5½oz) mango, cut into 1cm
  (½in) cubes

1 medium avocado, cut into 1cm
  (½in) cubes

2 radishes or 1 turnip, finely sliced
  (optional)

¼–½ jalapeño chilli or hot green
  or red chilli, according to taste,
  finely sliced

½ teaspoon salt

a small handful of coriander leaves,
  roughly chopped

juice of 2 limes

Per serving
7.4g net carbs, 3g fibre,
13.9g protein, 8.1g fat, 164kcal

This Peruvian classic can be a simple mixture of lime juice, chilli and salt poured over fish and fruit. It appears to "cook" the fish in minutes, turning it from translucent to opaque, but what actually happens is that the proteins are denatured by the acid of the citrus fruit, which gives the fish a cooked texture.

As the fish is not cooked using any heat, it is important that it is "sushi-grade" fresh and safe to eat, or that it has been commercially frozen at -20°C (-4°F) as this kills any possible parasites. This is difficult to do in a domestic freezer, but a good fishmonger can do this for you and a lot of fish sold in supermarkets has been previously frozen. Alternatively, use cooked prawns in this recipe, as they are just as good.

Usually fruit such as grapes, peach or mango is added to ceviche to give a welcome sweetness after the punchy citrus and salt. Lime is sometimes replaced with acidic passion fruit to do the same job. Tropical fruits are high in carbs and therefore usually avoided in our recipes, but we have used a minimal quantity here. Any remaining mango can be cut into cubes and frozen for use another day.

I like to add something crunchy like radishes or turnips but it's not strictly necessary. To get ahead, stop after mixing the fish, fruit and vegetables together and keep the bowl in the fridge, covered, for up to a day. Add the salt and lime just before serving. Do taste your chilli so that you know how much to add. It is disappointing to not have enough of a kick of heat or overpowering to have too much.

Soak the onions in cold water for 10 minutes to diminish their strength.

Gently mix the fish, mango, avocado, radishes, if using, and chilli together in a mixing bowl. Drain and add the onions.

Add the salt, coriander and lime juice and gently toss through. Taste and add salt as necessary.

Divide between serving dishes and serve straight away.

CREAMY WINE & GARLIC MUSSELS

L

SERVES 4

1kg (2lb 4oz) live mussels, scrubbed and beards removed (see intro)

2 tablespoons olive oil

3 garlic cloves, lightly crushed

100ml (3½fl oz) white wine (not too sweet)

25g (1oz) butter

100ml (3½fl oz) double cream

a handful of flat-leaf parsley, stems finely chopped, leaves torn

freshly ground black pepper

salt (optional)

Per serving
6.8g net carbs, 0g fibre,
31g protein, 29g fat, 425kcal

This dish always reminds me of holidays in France. Mussels are easy to cook at home and with a white or brown bread roll (pages 69 and 67), and a glass of dry, white wine, I feel like I have packed my bags and travelled.

When you buy fresh mussels or clams, check them carefully and discard any with cracked or broken shells. Rinse the mussels well in a bowl with several changes of water. Pull off the beards by holding the mussels, pointed end facing you, and pulling the beard towards you. Mussels should close if tapped on a hard surface; if any remain open, they are dead and should be discarded.

Put the mussels in a large pan over a medium heat. Add the olive oil, garlic, white wine and some black pepper, cover and cook for 5 minutes.

Add the butter and cream, re-cover and cook for a further 5 minutes. Discard any mussels that do not open. Taste the sauce; you probably don't need salt but add if necessary. If there is any grit at the bottom of the pan, pass the mussels and sauce through a sieve.

Serve the mussels in warm bowls topped with the parsley. Don't forget a spare bowl to put the empty shells in.

CREAMY COD & BROCCOLI MORNAY

SERVES 2

150g (5½oz) broccoli, cut into florets

100ml (3½fl oz) double cream

100ml (3½fl oz) just-boiled water

200g (7oz) skinless cod or haddock fillets

2 teaspoons cornflour

¼ teaspoon freshly grated nutmeg

75g (2¾oz) mature Cheddar cheese, coarsely grated

salt and freshly ground black pepper

Per serving
7.2g net carbs, 2.5g fibre,
31.2g protein, 34.7g fat, 475kcal

I remember eating boil-in-the-bag Cod Mornay in my teens; if only I had realized how easy it was to make, I would have done it myself rather than buying processed food. I have added broccoli to make it a deliciously satisfying one-pot supper.

Heat your grill as hot as it will go.

Put the broccoli into a pan of boiling water and cook for 6 minutes or until tender. Drain and transfer to a grill-proof dish.

Pour the cream and just-boiled water into a saucepan and cook over a medium heat. When the liquid is hot and gently bubbling, poach the fish, covered, for 6 minutes or until just cooked through. This will depend on the size of the fish pieces. Remove from the pan with a slotted spoon and put into the dish with the broccoli.

Mix the cornflour into 3 tablespoons of water and add this to the cream, then bring to the boil and stir until it thickens. Stir in the nutmeg and 50g (1¾oz) of the grated cheese, then taste and season accordingly. Pour the sauce over the fish, making sure it is covered. Pour it over the broccoli too, but it doesn't matter if the florets aren't completely covered as charred broccoli is wonderful.

Scatter over the remaining cheese and grill close to the heat source for 5 minutes or until bubbling and lightly browned.

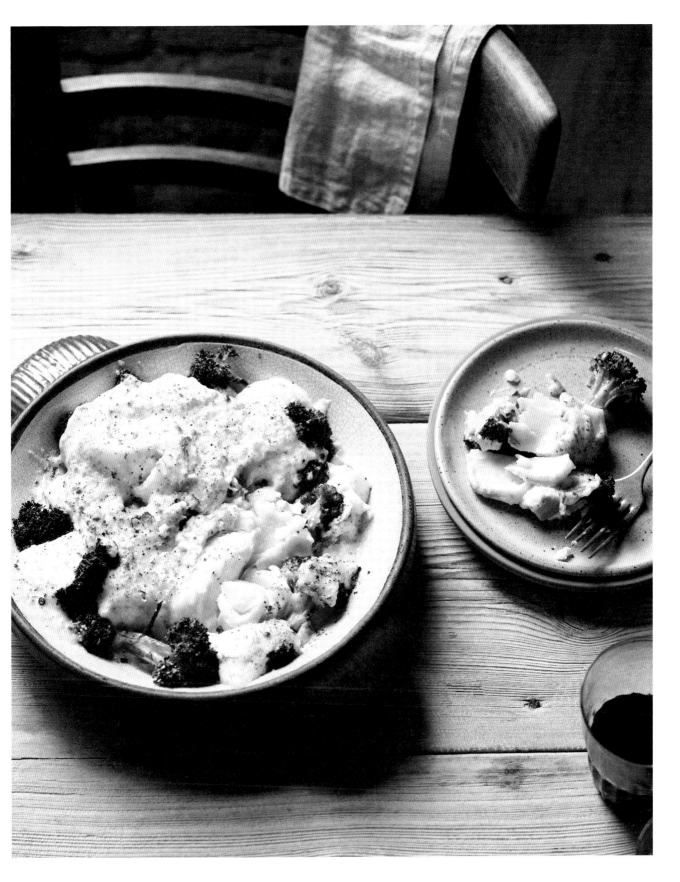

MEDITERRANEAN SARDINE BAKE

L
SERVES 4

200g (7oz) green beans, trimmed, or
  courgettes, cut into batons

1 small red pepper, cut into thin strips

1 small onion, finely sliced, or 3 spring
  onions, finely sliced

4 cans (84g/3oz drained weight per
  can) sardines or mackerel, drained

8 cherry tomatoes, halved

1 tablespoon capers, rinsed (optional)

1 fat garlic clove, finely sliced

4 tablespoons extra virgin olive oil
  (from the sardine cans or bottle)

1 teaspoon dried oregano

a pinch of chilli flakes or a little fresh
  chilli, finely chopped (optional)

salt and freshly ground black pepper

Per serving
9.7g net carbs, 4.6g fibre,
24.3g protein, 22.9g fat, 347kcal

Hot sardines scented with oregano, capers and chilli, this recipe takes me straight to Italy. This economical and flavourful dish couldn't be easier to put together – I rustle it up for a summer lunch outside or have it in half portions as a starter with salad leaves. Don't be put off by canned fish; they are just as nutritious as their fresh counterparts, but if you do have fresh sardines, you can use those instead, allowing 2 to 3 fish per person depending on their size.

Heat your grill as hot as it will go.

Preheat the oven to 200°C/180°C fan/400°F/gas mark 6.

Cook the green beans in boiling salted water for about 5 minutes until just tender. Drain and set aside.

Assemble the beans, red pepper, onion, sardines, tomatoes, capers and garlic in a large, ovenproof dish. Tuck the sardines between the beans and push the garlic into the vegetables so that it doesn't burn. Drizzle over the oil, then scatter over the oregano, chilli and some salt and pepper.

Bake for 30 minutes until the onions are starting to brown and the tomatoes have softened. Serve on warm plates.

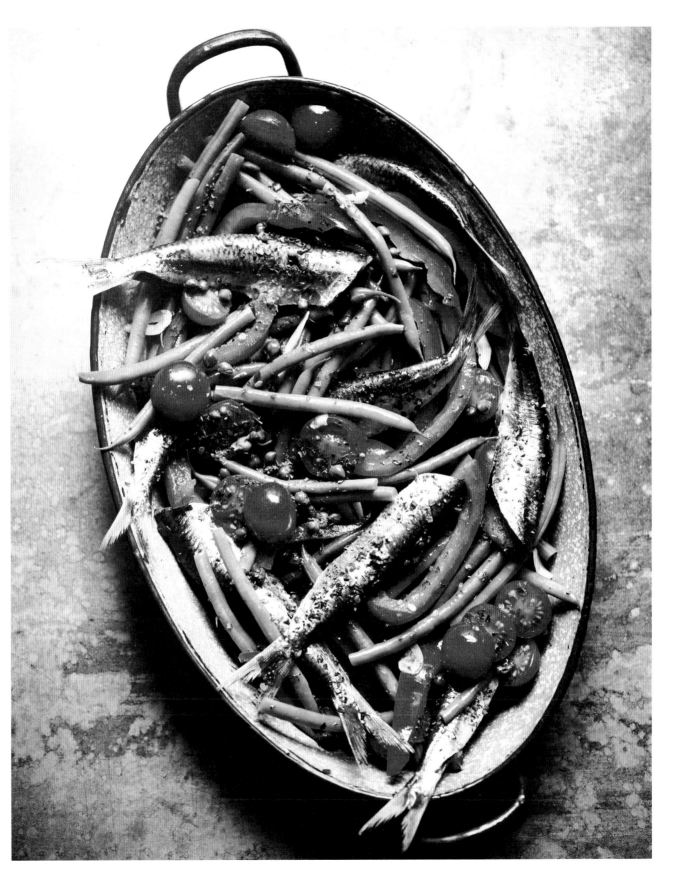

MISO SALMON & STIR-FRIED NOODLES

SERVES 2

20g (¾oz) fresh ginger, peeled and grated

1 garlic clove, grated

2 tablespoons white or red miso paste

1 teaspoon mirin or honey

2 skinless salmon fillets, weighing about 150g (5½oz) each

For the noodles

200g (7oz) konjac noodles

2 garlic cloves, finely sliced

15g (½oz) fresh ginger, peeled and cut into julienne

1 small, hot chilli, finely sliced

1 tablespoon ghee, olive oil or coconut oil, plus extra for greasing

100g (3½oz) leeks or 6 spring onions, cut into julienne

1 small red pepper, finely sliced

1 small courgette, ribboned

1 tablespoon soy sauce or tamari

2 teaspoons toasted sesame oil

2 teaspoons toasted white or black sesame seeds (optional)

½–1 teaspoon shichimi togarashi (optional)

Per serving
13g net carbs, 5.5g fibre,
41g protein, 35g fat, 551kcal

Miso adds a rich, salty, umami flavour to anything it touches. It comes in a paste and therefore lends itself to coating foods such as salmon, or mackerel if you prefer. If you need a hand on cutting techniques like the julienne, which means cutting into matchsticks, see www.thegoodkitchentable.com. This is an ideal dish to prepare in advance of a date night! Get everything chopped and ready while the fish marinates and in 15 minutes dinner will be served.

Mix the ginger, garlic, miso and mirin together and brush all over the salmon. Leave, covered, for 30 minutes or overnight. The flavour is more intense the longer you leave it.

Preheat the oven to 220°C/200°C fan/425°F/gas mark 7 and grease an ovenproof dish or baking tray.

Transfer the marinated salmon to the prepared tray and bake for 15 minutes or until it is firm to the touch and doesn't feel at all wobbly.

Meanwhile, rinse the noodles thoroughly in plenty of cold water and drain.

Stir-fry the garlic, ginger and chilli in the ghee in a medium frying pan over a medium–high heat for 1 minute. Stir in the leeks, red pepper and courgette, then add the drained noodles, soy sauce and toasted sesame oil. Stir through, put on the lid and cook for 3 minutes or until the courgettes have wilted. Taste the noodles and add more soy sauce as necessary.

Divide the stir-fry between 2 warm bowls. Lay the salmon on top and scatter over the sesame seeds and shichimi togarashi, if using.

FISH & COCONUT CURRY

SERVES 6

4 tablespoons ghee, coconut oil or
   extra virgin olive oil

2 red onions, roughly chopped

1 green bird's eye chilli

2 teaspoons Kashmiri chilli powder

2 fat garlic cloves, grated

50g (1¾oz) fresh ginger, grated

1 teaspoon salt

½ teaspoon freshly ground
   black pepper

½ teaspoon ground turmeric

½ teaspoon black mustard seeds

400g (400ml) can of full-fat
   coconut milk

10 fresh curry leaves, washed,
   or 20 dried curry leaves

1kg (2lb 4oz) skinless huss, cod or
   similar white fish, or salmon, cut
   into 5cm (2in) pieces

a small handful of coriander leaves,
   to serve

Per serving
12g net carbs, 2.8g fibre,
36g protein, 37g fat, 532kcal

I was interested to try different fish in this recipe loosely based on a Keralan molee and delighted to find huss, which is also known as dogfish or rock. It is inexpensive, local to our shores in the UK and robust enough to be cooked and enjoyed in this glorious golden bath of coconut curry. Look out for local, sustainable firm white fish or use seafood instead. Try to find fragrant fresh curry leaves if you can, they make all the difference and can be frozen. If you are using dried leaves, add an extra ten to bump up the flavour. Serve with Cauli rice (page 93) or steamed broccoli.

Heat the ghee in a large frying pan or heavy-based saucepan over a medium–high heat. Add the onions and cook for 7–10 minutes, stirring frequently, until soft and starting to brown. Add the chilli, chilli powder, garlic, ginger, seasoning, turmeric and mustard seeds and fry for a further 5 minutes.

Pour in the coconut milk, bring to the boil, then reduce the heat to a simmer. Blend the sauce with a stick blender (or leave as it is). Add the curry leaves. At this point the sauce can be left until you are almost ready to eat, as the fish should be added at the last moment to avoid it breaking up.

Add the fish and cook for about 5 minutes, covered and stirring occasionally, or until the fish is just cooked through.

Taste the sauce and adjust the seasoning as necessary. Serve straight away in warm bowls topped with the coriander leaves.

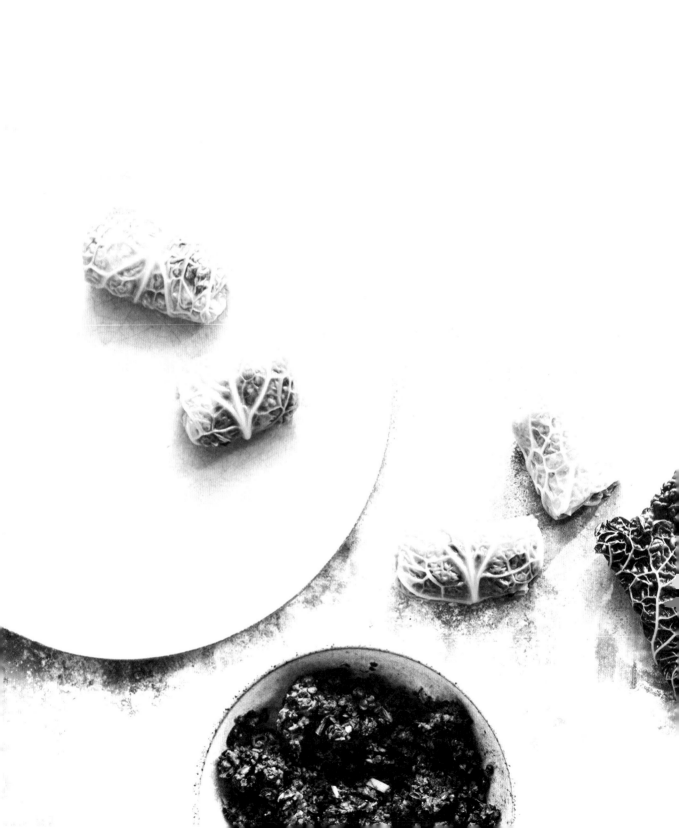

VEG

SMOKY, STUFFED MEDITERRANEAN PEPPERS

L

SERVES 4

4 medium red, green or
    yellow peppers

1 large leek, finely chopped

1 fat garlic clove, finely chopped

4 tablespoons extra virgin olive oil

150g (5½oz) cauliflower, riced (see
    page 93)

100g (3½oz) feta cheese, crumbled
    (optional)

50g (1¾oz) Parmesan or Grana
    Padano, finely grated

20g (¾oz) flat-leaf parsley, finely
    chopped, plus extra sprigs to serve

2 heaped teaspoons smoked sweet
    paprika, plus extra as necessary

60g (2¼oz) sun-dried tomatoes,
    roughly chopped

12 cherry tomatoes, halved

100g (3½oz) thick Greek yogurt

salt and freshly ground black pepper

Per serving
15g net carbs, 8.1g fibre,
14g protein, 29g fat, 399kcal

This recipe is for our wonderful vegetarian friend Anne Hudson who helps me test recipes. She is often disappointed by vegetarian offerings, so inspired by our Mediterranean travels together, we invented this dish full of colour and flavour, from the Spanish smoked paprika to Greek feta and Italian Parmesan and sun-dried tomatoes.

Slice the tops off the peppers about 2cm (¾in) from the stalks; they can be chopped into a salad another day. Discard the pith and seeds. Check the peppers will stand upright; if not, cut a small sliver off the bottoms, making sure not to make a hole, and stand them in an ovenproof dish or on a baking tray.

Preheat the oven to 200°C/180°C fan/400°F/gas mark 6.

To make the stuffing, fry the leek and garlic in 3 tablespoons of the oil and 2 tablespoons of water over a medium heat for about 7 minutes or until soft. Add the cauliflower and some seasoning and stir through. Cook, covered, for a further 5–7 minutes or until the cauliflower is just tender. Tip into a bowl and leave to cool for a few minutes. Add the cheeses, parsley, paprika and sun-dried tomatoes and stir to combine. Taste the stuffing and adjust with seasoning or add more paprika as you like.

Fill the peppers with the stuffing and top each one with the halved cherry tomatoes. Drizzle over the remaining tablespoon of oil and add a little more seasoning. Cook the peppers for 35–45 minutes or until tender – it will depend on their size. Any leftover stuffing can be added to scrambled eggs or a frittata another day.

Serve the peppers warm in a serving dish with a swirl of the cooking juices over the top and a sprig of parsley, with the yogurt on the side.

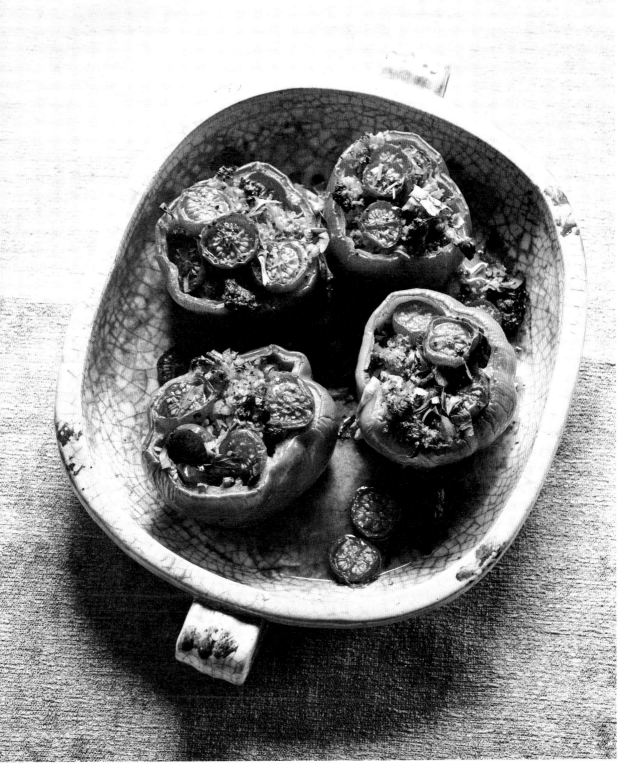

SPICED AUBERGINE WITH TOMATOES & CRISPY ONIONS ON FETA CREAM

L

SERVES 4

2 medium aubergines

2 teaspoons harissa or chipotle paste

2 tablespoons Greek yogurt

3 tablespoons extra virgin olive oil

1 red pepper, cut into 8 long wedges

a handful of flat-leaf parsley or coriander, stems finely chopped and leaves roughly chopped

salt and freshly ground black pepper

For the crispy onions

1 medium onion, very thinly sliced into half-moons

2 tablespoons extra virgin olive oil

For the feta cream

100g (3½oz) feta or goat's cheese

200g (7oz) thick Greek or strained yogurt

Per serving
14.5g net carbs, 4.4g fibre,
9.3g protein, 23.7g fat, 313kcal

This pretty dish is lovely on its own for lunch or as part of a buffet with other salads. You can also use the harissa paste in the Chorizo & pepper cauli rice on page 94. Serve with soft-boiled eggs for extra protein.

Preheat the oven to 200°C/180°C fan/400°F/gas mark 6.

Cut the aubergines into long wedges about 3cm (1¼in) at the widest part. Then cut across but not through the wedges in a series of shallow cuts about 1.5cm (⅝in) deep and 1.5cm (⅝in) apart. Put the aubergines into a roasting dish.

Stir the harissa into the yogurt and add 2 tablespoons of the oil. Mix together and brush over the aubergines. Put the red pepper into the baking dish and drizzle over the remaining tablespoon of olive oil. Scatter a little salt and pepper over all the vegetables. Bake for 20–25 minutes or until the aubergines are lightly browned and cooked through.

Meanwhile, cook the onion in the oil in a frying pan over a medium heat for at least 10–15 minutes. Stir frequently and season to taste while the onion cooks. Remove from the heat when browned and crisp.

Prepare the feta cream by mashing the cheese and yogurt together with a fork. Spread the feta cream over a plate and top with the roast aubergines, pepper, crispy onions and the oil they were cooked in. Scatter over the herbs just before serving.

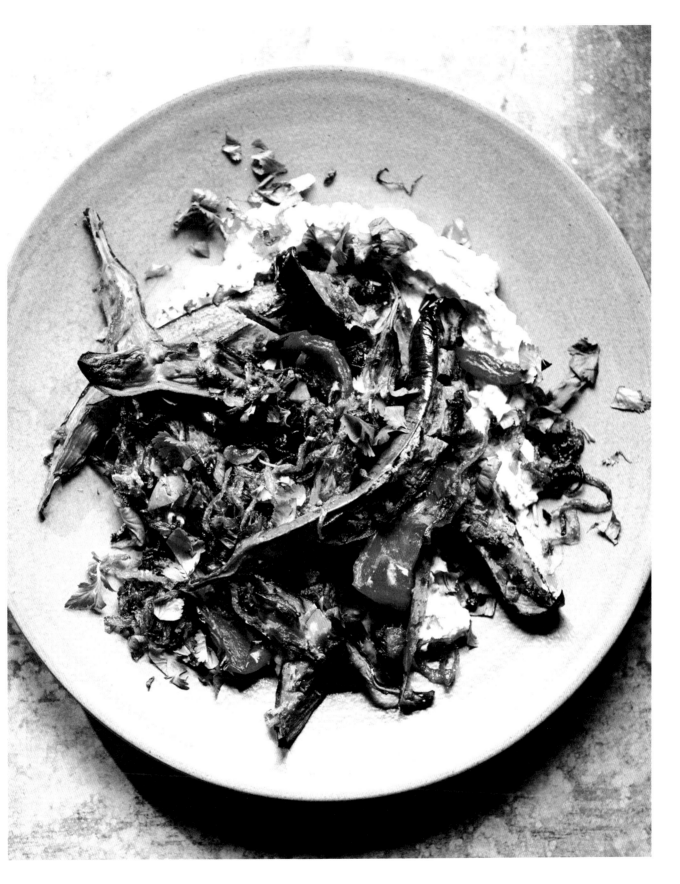

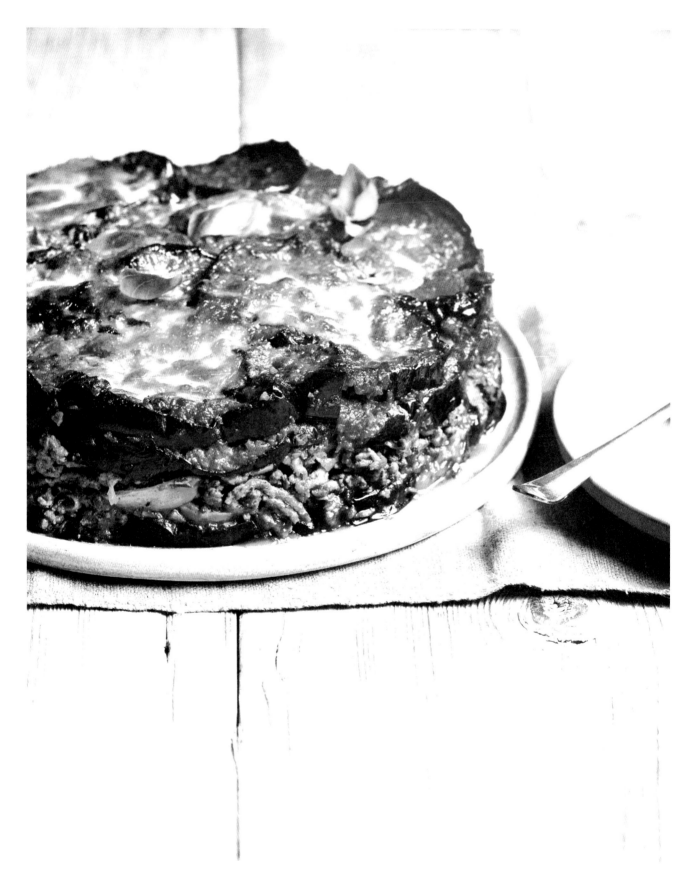

AUBERGINE PARMIGIANA

L   as it is

G   with mince

SERVES 8

4 tablespoons extra virgin olive oil,
   for greasing and brushing

5 medium aubergines (approx.
   1.2kg/2lb 11oz), cut into 1.5cm
   (⅝in) slices

2 x 125g (4½oz) balls of buffalo
   mozzarella

1 x quantity of Classic Italian tomato
   sauce (page 88)

1 x quantity of Quick stir-fried lamb
   mince (page 125)

10g broad basil leaves

50g (1¾oz) Parmesan cheese,
   finely grated

salt and freshly ground black pepper

Per serving
21g net carbs, 8.8g fibre,
11.7g protein, 23.9g fat, 360kcal

with lamb mince
21g net carbs, 8.8g fibre,
27.2g protein, 26.1g fat, 447kcal

This classic Italian recipe is inherently low carb; however, the aubergines are often coated in flour or breadcrumbs and then deep-fried. Here is my lighter, simpler version with roast aubergines and made in a cake tin so that it makes an impressive vegetarian or meat-eater's main course. It's perfect for a supper with family or friends, or for batch cooking, as it lasts well in the fridge or can be frozen.

Preheat the oven to 240°C/220°C fan/475°F/gas mark 9 and grease a 23cm (9in) loose-bottomed cake tin and a baking tray with olive oil.

Lay the aubergine slices on the prepared baking tray. Brush the tops with olive oil and season lightly with salt and pepper. Roast the aubergines for about 20 minutes or until lightly browned. Remove any thinner ones from the tray if they start to burn before the others are ready.

Cut or tear the mozzarella into pieces and drain in a sieve while you prepare the aubergines.

Purée the tomato sauce with a stick blender or in a food processor if you like a smooth sauce.

Remove the aubergines from the oven and set aside. Reduce the oven temperature to 200°C/180°C fan/400°F/gas mark 6.

Lay one-third of the aubergine slices, tightly packed, over the base of the prepared cake tin. Top with one-third of the tomato sauce, mince, if using, basil leaves, mozzarella and Parmesan. Repeat twice more, finishing with a layer of cheese. Put the cake tin into a roasting dish to catch any leakage and bake for 30 minutes or until the cheese is golden brown.

Remove from the oven and leave to rest for 15 minutes. Use a dinner knife to loosen the parmigiana from the tin around the edge. Carefully remove the cake ring and use a thin spatula to slide the parmigiana on to a serving plate with a rim (as the juices can leak out). Cut into wedges with a serrated knife and enjoy.

GIORGIO'S MOUTABAL

U

SERVES 6

2 medium aubergines (approx.
1kg/2lb 4oz)

100g (3½oz) Greek yogurt

1 small garlic clove, grated or
finely diced

2 tablespoons tahini

juice of 1 lemon

½–1 teaspoon salt

freshly ground black pepper

To serve

1 tablespoon extra virgin olive oil

½ teaspoon paprika or sumac
(optional)

Per serving
2.6g net carbs, 2.2g fibre,
3.7g protein, 7.2g fat, 94kcal

Our friend Amal Al Qahtani used to make this for our son Giorgio when she came to stay with us from Kuwait; if we weren't careful, he would eat the whole bowl before we got a chance to have any. At home, Amal uses a gas hob to blister the skin of the aubergines. I have used our barbecue or got our boys to hold the aubergines with long tongs and burnt them with a cook's blowtorch. Now, I just use a hot grill, which is a little less dramatic but works just as well to achieve a smoky flavour.

Heat the grill to its hottest setting.

While the grill is heating, prick the aubergines and put them under the grill as close as you can to the heat. Cook them for about 15–20 minutes until wrinkled and blistered all over, to the point where they are starting to collapse, turning them using tongs every 5 minutes.

Meanwhile, put the yogurt, garlic, tahini, lemon juice and seasoning into a mixing bowl and stir to combine.

Remove the aubergines from the grill and set aside to cool. When cool to the touch, peel off the skins and lay the flesh on a chopping board. Chop it to a pulp with a large knife and pour away any water that comes out. Put it into the bowl with the yogurt mixture, stir to combine and taste for seasoning and lemon.

Transfer the moutabal to a serving bowl and pour over the oil. Dust it with paprika or sumac and serve. The dip will hold in the fridge for a day or two but always decorate just before serving with raw vegetable sticks or the Super seed crackers on page 73.

TAMARI MUSHROOM BOWL

(G) with added protein
SERVES 2

For the mushrooms

1 tablespoon tamari or dark or light
    soy sauce

3 tablespoons extra virgin olive oil

200g (7oz) chestnut mushrooms,
    sliced

freshly ground black pepper

For the tomato, celery & chilli salad

150g (5½oz) cherry tomatoes, halved

1 celery stick with leaves,
    roughly chopped

1 green chilli, finely sliced

1 tablespoon extra virgin olive oil

pinch of salt

For the avocado mash

1 ripe, medium avocado

1 tablespoon lemon juice

1 garlic clove, finely chopped
    (optional)

a small handful of coriander or
    flat-leaf parsley, finely chopped
    (optional)

This is a delicious light lunch or a side dish. To bump up the protein, add strips of cooked chicken, soft-boiled eggs, tofu or a handful of the Spicy seed crunch from page 150. See the photo on page 7 for inspiration.

Preheat the oven to 220°C/200°C fan/425°F/gas mark 7 and line a roasting tray with baking parchment.

Mix the tamari and oil together in a mixing bowl. Add the mushrooms to the bowl, give it a few twists of black pepper and toss through. Spread the mushrooms out in the roasting tray and roast for 20 minutes or until cooked through and any water has evaporated.

To make the salad, mix all the ingredients together in a bowl and season to taste.

To make the avocado mash, use a fork to mash the avocado flesh in a bowl with the lemon juice, garlic and coriander, if using.

Divide the three recipe elements between 2 bowls and serve straight away.

Per serving
of mushrooms
2.7g net carbs, 1.1g fibre, 4g protein, 20.6g fat, 206kcal

of tomato, celery & chilli salad
2.3g net carbs, 1.2g fibre, 0.8g protein, 6.9g fat, 76kcal

of avocado mash
1.7g net carbs, 4.6g fibre, 1.4g protein, 10.5g fat, 115kcal

of all three salads
6.7g net carbs, 6.9g fibre, 6.2g protein, 38g fat, 397kcal

RAINBOWL

Excuse the pun but this was called A rainbow bowl of salad originally and, over time, it became shortened to Rainbowl, but I'm sure you realize it isn't a bowl of rainwater! As Dr David Unwin says, "ban the beige" from your plate, so here's a big bowl of colour!

To get all the nutrients and a variety of textures in your Rainbowl, choose one from each of the categories below:

Protein: 2 eggs, cooked meat or chicken livers, tuna, salmon, sardines, tofu, nuts, hemp seeds, pumpkin seeds, black or edamame beans, quinoa or the Spicy seed crunch.
Healthy fat: olives, extra virgin olive oil, avocado slices, Spicy avocado salad (page 162), Avocado mash (page 149), nuts, One-minute mayonnaise (page 179), soured cream, Giorgio's moutabal (page 148) or Greek yogurt
Get your greens: approx. 20g (¾oz) raw chopped kale or baby spinach leaves, courgette ribbons, lettuce, rocket
Red: tomatoes, strips of pepper, red cabbage, carrot, beetroot
Add a crunch: shaved turnips, radishes, live sauerkraut or kimchi, apple, or use the Super slaw (page 166) or the Pickled red cabbage (page 152)
Dressings: Classic vinaigrette, Golden or Miso dressing (page 180)

DRY-FRIED HALLOUMI

These moreish slices are great to fry up quickly and add to salads, so perfect for the Rainbowl or to have with a side dish.

L   SERVES 4
250g (9oz) halloumi, cut into 10 slices

Dry-fry the halloumi in a non-stick frying pan. Water sometimes comes out of the cheese, so allow this to evaporate. Turn the cheese when it is browned and fry the other side. Use straight away or the cheese becomes firm and squeaky again quickly.

Per slice
0.5g net carbs, 0g fibre, 5.3g protein, 6.5g fat, 81kcal

SPICY SEED CRUNCH

Use a variety of seeds for this recipe but try to include pumpkin and hemp as they contain the most protein. I sometimes add in black onion seeds (nigella) or toasted cumin seeds to alter the flavour. All these seeds contain healthy fats but are also high in calories, so make sure you don't mindlessly snack on them. They are part of a meal rather than something to be eaten in between.

L   SERVES 6
50g (1¾oz) pumpkin seeds
50g (1¾oz) sunflower seeds
25g (1oz) hemp seeds
50g (1¾oz) sesame seeds, flaxseed or chia seeds
1 tablespoon extra virgin olive, coconut or avocado oil
1 tablespoon tamari
pinch of something hot, such as chilli powder, cayenne or Aleppo pepper

Preheat the oven to 220°C/200°C fan/425°F/ gas mark 7 and line a baking tray with baking parchment.

Toss the seeds with the remaining ingredients in a small bowl. Tip on to the prepared baking tray and spread out with the back of a spoon. Bake for 6 minutes or until the seeds are toasted and crunchy.

Remove from the oven and set aside to cool. Use the parchment to shoot them into a jar or similar container and use within a week.

Per serving
2.2g net carbs, 2.6g fibre, 8.9g protein, 19.8g fat, 216kcal

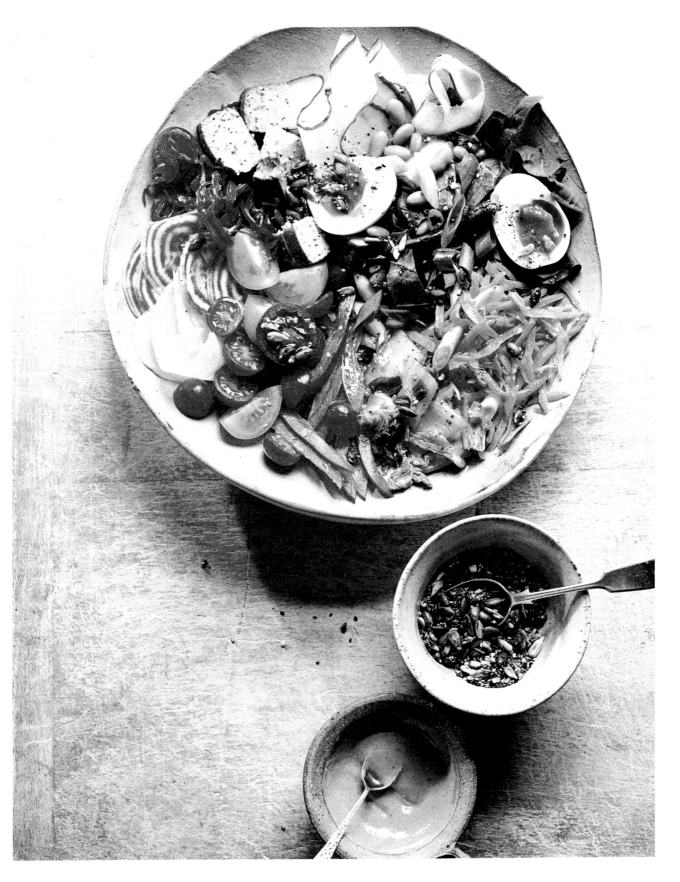

PICKLED RED CABBAGE

This deep purple salad is sweet, sour and spicy. It keeps well in the fridge, so can be on hand to add to a Rainbowl with any of the salads, with soft-boiled eggs and it is particularly good with the Aquafaba mayonnaise and the Golden tahini & turmeric dressing on pages 179 and 180.

L

SERVES 4

300g (10½oz) red cabbage

250ml (9fl oz) cider vinegar

2 teaspoons honey or 1 heaped tablespoon erythritol (optional)

1–2 teaspoons salt, to taste

a thumb-sized piece of fresh ginger, peeled and finely sliced (optional)

½–1 finely sliced hot chilli or a pinch of chilli flakes (optional)

Discard the end of the woody core of the cabbage and the outer leaves if soft. Use a food processor with the slicing attachment, a sharp knife or a mandoline to shred the cabbage into thin ribbons.

Put the vinegar, honey or erythritol, 1 teaspoon of salt, 250ml (9fl oz) water and additional flavourings, if using, into a saucepan and bring to the boil. Add the red cabbage and bring to the boil again. Remove from the heat and leave to cool to room temperature.

Use straight away, removing the cabbage from the pickling liquid, or transfer the cabbage and the liquid to a container such as a Mason jar. It can be stored in the fridge, once cool, for up to 2 weeks. As time goes by the flavour will develop and the vinegar will mellow.

Per serving
with honey
8.4g net carbs, 1.6g fibre, 1.1g protein, 0.1g fat, 47kcal

with erythritol
5.3g net carbs, 1.6g fibre, 1.2g protein, 0.2g fat, 40kcal

CELERY & STILTON SOUP

L
SERVES 6

1 leek (approx. 150g/5½oz) or onion,
  finely chopped

400g (14oz) celery, roughly chopped,
  reserving a few leaves to serve

50g (1¾oz) butter

1 litre (1¾ pints) warm chicken, meat
  or vegetable stock

200g (7oz) Stilton cheese, rind on
  and roughly chopped

salt and freshly ground black pepper

To serve (optional)
celery leaves
a little freshly grated nutmeg
a drizzle of extra virgin olive oil

Per serving
3.3g net carbs, 1.3g fibre,
8.7g protein, 18.6g fat, 216kcal

We love to make this soup and I have often served it to people who claim not to like blue cheese – it doesn't taste overwhelmingly of it, more the cheese gives it a savoury bite. Enjoy it as a first course, a light meal or with a slice of one of the low-carb breads in the book. If you don't have Stilton, use any blue cheese or a mature firm cheese instead. In case you are wondering, Stilton is usually vegetarian.

Gently fry the leek and celery in the butter with some seasoning in a large saucepan, covered, for 10 minutes.

Add the warm stock and Stilton and bring to the boil. Remove the pan from the heat and blend the soup with a stick blender or liquidizer until smooth. Return the pan to warm over a high heat and season to taste. Serve straight away as it is or with one of the suggested toppings.

SAAG-STYLE KALE & PANEER

L   as it is

G   with chapatti

SERVES 4 AS A MAIN
OR 6 AS A SIDE

500g (1lb 2oz) kale, Swiss chard,
   spinach, spring greens or
   cabbage, stems removed and
   finely chopped

2 tablespoons ghee or 1 tablespoon
   butter and 1 tablespoon olive oil

200g (7oz) paneer, cut into 1.5cm
   (⅝in) or bite-sized cubes

3 fat garlic cloves, finely chopped
   or grated

1 hot green or red chilli, finely
   chopped, or 1 teaspoon chilli flakes

1 teaspoon cumin seeds

1 teaspoon ground turmeric

120ml (4fl oz) double cream

salt and freshly ground black pepper

Per serving
between 6
2.5g net carbs, 3.4g fibre,
10g protein, 25.6g fat, 286kcal

between 4
3.8g net carbs, 5g fibre,
15.1g protein, 38.4g fat, 429kcal

This is traditionally made with spinach but I experimented recently with some leftover curly kale. It worked brilliantly and then our friend Preeti Gohil said she frequently makes it with a selection of greens, so now it is made with whatever I have in the fridge or garden, including cavolo nero, Swiss chard, spinach, sprout tops, spring greens, curly kale or Savoy cabbage.

Boil the kale in salted water for 10 minutes or until soft. Drain and set aside.

Heat the ghee in a deep frying pan or saucepan over a medium–high heat and fry the paneer on all sides until golden brown. Use a slotted spoon to remove the paneer from the pan and set aside.

Add the garlic, chilli and spices to the pan with some salt and pepper and fry over a medium heat for 1 minute, making sure that the garlic doesn't burn.

Add the drained kale to the pan and stir through for a few minutes until hot. Add the cream and stir again to heat through. Taste and adjust the seasoning. Serve straight away or keep and reheat. It will keep well in the fridge for up to 3 days or in the freezer for up to 3 months.

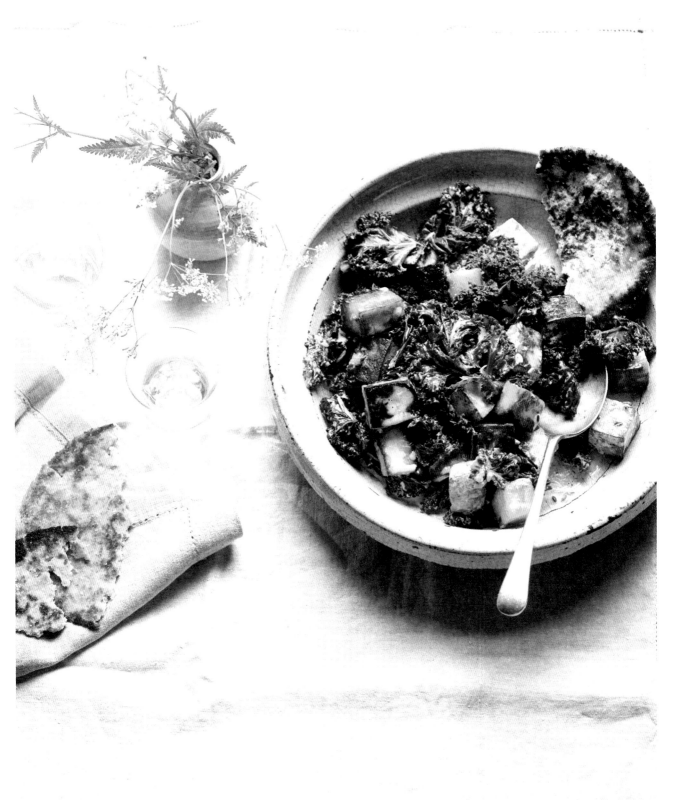

VIBRANT VEGETABLE KORMA

L   as it is
 with paneer
SERVES 6

5 tablespoons ghee or
   2½ tablespoons extra virgin olive
   oil and 2½ tablespoons butter

2 medium onions, finely sliced

700g (1lb 9oz) mixture of low-carb
   vegetables, such as green beans,
   sprouts, broccoli, cauliflower,
   mangetout, courgettes and/or
   peppers

250g (9oz) Greek yogurt

½ teaspoon ground turmeric

1 teaspoon ground coriander

1 teaspoon Kashmiri or mild red
   chilli powder

2 teaspoons curry powder

40g (1½oz) blanched almonds or
   cashews, soaked overnight,
   then drained

200g (7oz) paneer, cut into cut into
   1.5cm (⅝in) or bite-sized cubes,
   (optional)

a thumb-sized cinnamon stick

5 green cardamom pods,
   lightly crushed

1 black cardamom pod (optional)

6 cloves

1 teaspoon freshly ground
   black pepper

1 bay leaf

1 small hot green or red chilli, split
   almost in two, or 1 teaspoon hot
   chilli powder (optional)

2 teaspoons finely grated ginger

2 fat garlic cloves, finely grated

I have tried many ways to make a delicious, creamy low-carb korma over the years and am so happy with this version. I've added nuts for extra protein since this is a vegetable curry. The nuts are best soaked overnight to soften them, but I have to confess that at times I have forgotten to soak them, and the curry was still creamy and gorgeous. If you don't have blanched almonds, brown ones with skin are fine. If you don't have a powerful food processor to blend the almonds, you can use ground almonds instead and slice the onions by hand.

I use low-carb vegetables, such as green beans, sprouts, broccoli, cauliflower, mangetout, courgettes, peppers or whatever we have in the garden or the fridge. To keep the cost down, you can use frozen beans or vegetables.

Since nutritionist Jenny Phillips suggests we eat 20–30g (¾–1oz) protein at every meal, you can see that the purely vegetable-based curry is low in this respect. I have, therefore, given the option of adding paneer, which will give you a more substantial meal or you could serve the curry with soft-boiled eggs (allow 2 per person) or with the Saag-style kale & paneer on page 154.

Heat 2 tablespoons of the ghee in a heavy-based pan over a medium–high heat and fry the onions, covered, for 10 minutes or until deeply browned, stirring frequently.

Meanwhile, cut the vegetables into bite-sized pieces and set aside. Whisk together the yogurt, turmeric, ground coriander, chilli and curry powders in a bowl and set aside.

When the onions are ready, transfer them to a bowl to cool. Keep the pan.

Once the onions have cooled a little, transfer them to a blender with the drained almonds and 100ml (3½fl oz) fresh water and blend to form a thick paste.

Heat the remaining 3 tablespoons of ghee in the pan that you used to cook the onions over a medium–low heat. Add the paneer, if using, and lightly brown on most sides. Add the cinnamon stick, green and black cardamom pods, cloves, black pepper and bay leaf. Sauté for a minute or two or until you can smell their fragrance. Then add the chilli, ginger and garlic and fry for a further 30 seconds.

250ml (9fl oz) just-boiled water

2 teaspoons garam masala (optional)

a handful of coriander,
    roughly chopped

salt, to taste

Per serving
10g net carbs, 5.4g fibre,
8.7g protein, 18g fat, 247kcal

with paneer
12g net carbs, 5.4g fibre,
24g protein, 36g fat, 482kcal

Now add the vegetables with the just-boiled water and stir through. Bring to the boil, then reduce the heat to a simmer and partially cover the pan. Depending on your choice of vegetables, you can leave the lid off to reduce the sauce if it is watery or have it completely covered if dry. Stir in the spiced yogurt, onion paste, and 1 teaspoon of salt and reduce the heat to medium–low. Cook for 15–20 minutes or until the vegetables are cooked through.

Remove from heat and stir in the garam masala and fresh coriander. If you are reheating the curry, always leave this last step until just before you serve. The curry keeps in the fridge for up to 3 days or freezes for up to 3 months.

SIU MAI

L
SERVES 4 AS A STARTER
OR 2 AS A MAIN

200g (7oz) Savoy or white cabbage

tamari or dark soy sauce, for dipping

5g (⅛oz) chives, finely chopped, or
    2 teaspoons toasted sesame seeds

For the stuffing

260g (9½oz) cooked Puy lentils,
    drained, or pork mince or
    minced prawns

2 spring onions, very finely chopped

20g (¾oz) fresh ginger, peeled
    and grated

2 fat garlic cloves, grated

1 small green or red Thai chilli, finely
    chopped, or a pinch of chilli flakes

1 egg white

2 teaspoons tamari or dark soy sauce

5g (⅛oz) chives, finely chopped

Per serving
made with lentils
12.6g net carbs, 5.2g fibre,
7.6g protein, 0.4g fat, 100kcal

made with pork
3.7g net carbs, 1.9g fibre,
18.1g protein, 9.4g fat, 175kcal

These are the typical little pork- or prawn-stuffed dim sum that are served in bamboo steamers in Chinese restaurants. Usually, the filling is wrapped in thin wheat-based wonton wrappers; however, we have created the same delicious recipe using cabbage leaves. They are easy to make and can be vegetarian depending on the filling. You can use a food processor to blitz the ingredients together for the stuffing, otherwise finely chop or grate the ingredients. The Siu mai can be made a day before you need them and kept in the fridge. Cook them just before serving. They make an ideal starter for four, or enjoy them as a main meal for two. (See pages 140–141 to see how they are made.)

Boil a large saucepan of water, big enough to hold the cabbage leaves. Cut the leaves away from the tough central stem of the cabbage, leaving each one whole. Now blanch the cabbage leaves in the boiling water for 2 minutes. They will float to the top so gently push them down as they boil. Use tongs to remove them from the water and lay them over a colander to drip dry and cool. I usually rest them around the edge and on the base of the colander, so they are not on top of one another. I then put the colander on the draining area of the sink, so the water runs away.

Make a paste for the stuffing by whizzing all the ingredients together in a food processor (in which case you only need to roughly chop the ingredients) or combine them together in a bowl with a spoon or your hands.

Now, take the cabbage leaves and prepare to get stuffing. Pat each one dry with kitchen paper or a tea towel and trim away any tough stems by holding the knife at an angle to slice off part of the stem. This will allow the leaf to fold but ensure the filling doesn't leak out.

Put a walnut-sized ball of stuffing in the centre of a leaf, on top of the stem. Fold in the sides and roll the cabbage leaf up from the nearest side to the farthest. You should have a neat, tight roll; place this in a steamer basket. Repeat with the remaining leaves and stuffing.

Steam the siu mai for 10–15 minutes or until cooked through and the filling is firm to the touch. Use tongs to remove each one and cut in half lengthways. Stand them up on a warm plate and serve them with the tamari for dipping. Scatter over the chives or toasted sesame seeds just before serving.

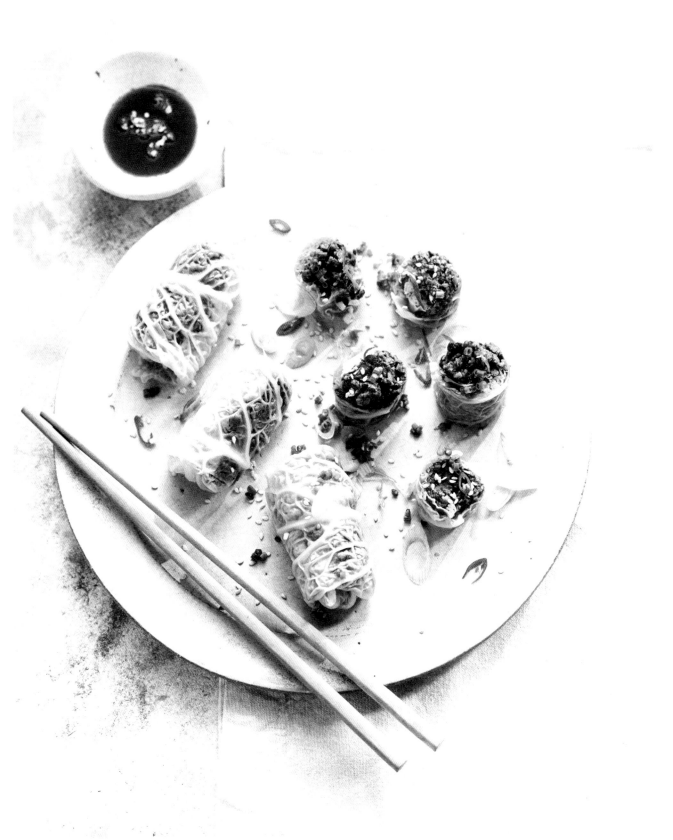

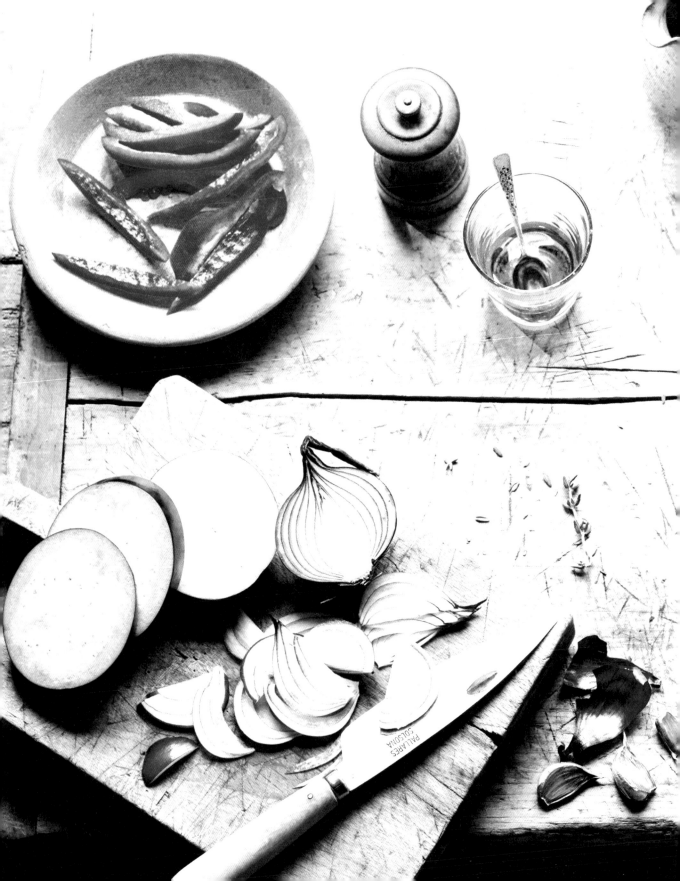

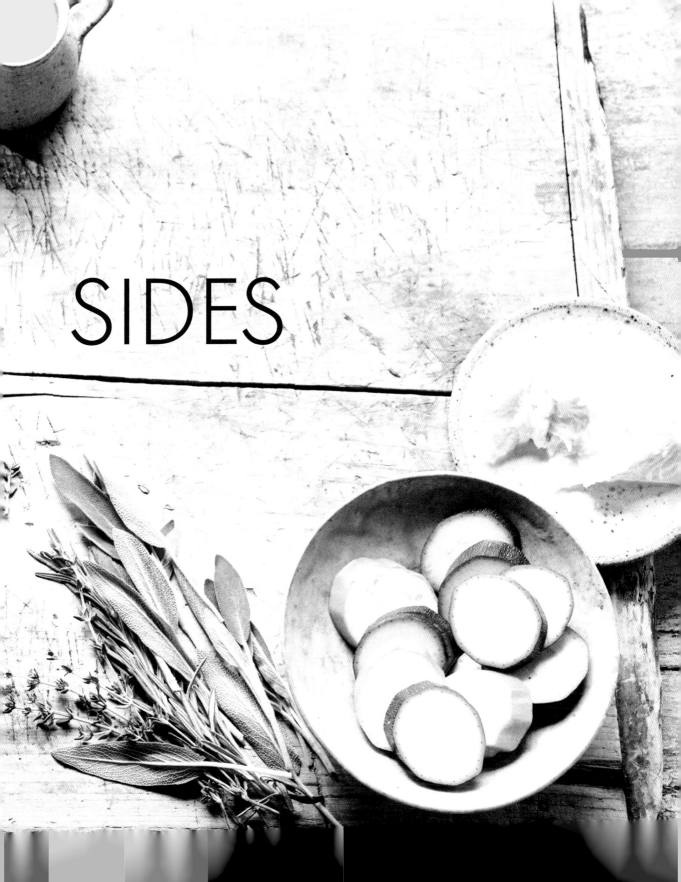

SIDES

SPICY AVOCADO SALAD

L

SERVES 4

3 spring onions or 1 small shallot, finely chopped

300g tomatoes, roughly chopped

1 celery stick, plus celery leaves, roughly chopped

2 avocados, diced into bite-sized cubes

juice of 1 lime or ½ lemon

1 red, green, orange or yellow pepper, cut into 3cm (1¼in) dice

¼–½ green or red chilli, finely chopped and added according to taste

4 tablespoons extra virgin olive oil

a small handful (approx. 15g/½oz) of coriander leaves, stalks finely chopped

salt and freshly ground black pepper

2 little gem lettuces, to serve

Per serving
7.7g net carbs, 9.1g fibre,
4g protein, 24.7g fat, 282kcal

This super-colourful salad is perfect with grilled salmon, steak, or feta cheese, or if you are at the higher end of the CarbScale (see page 24), add in a can of chickpeas or black beans.

Soak the spring onions in a bowl of cold water for 10 minutes to dilute their strength.

Drain the onions and put these into a serving bowl with the remaining ingredients, except the lettuces, and toss through gently.

Cut off the ends of the lettuces and pull the leaves apart. Stand them up at the edge of a serving bowl or serve alongside so they can be used to scoop up the salad. Give it an extra twist of black pepper and serve straight away.

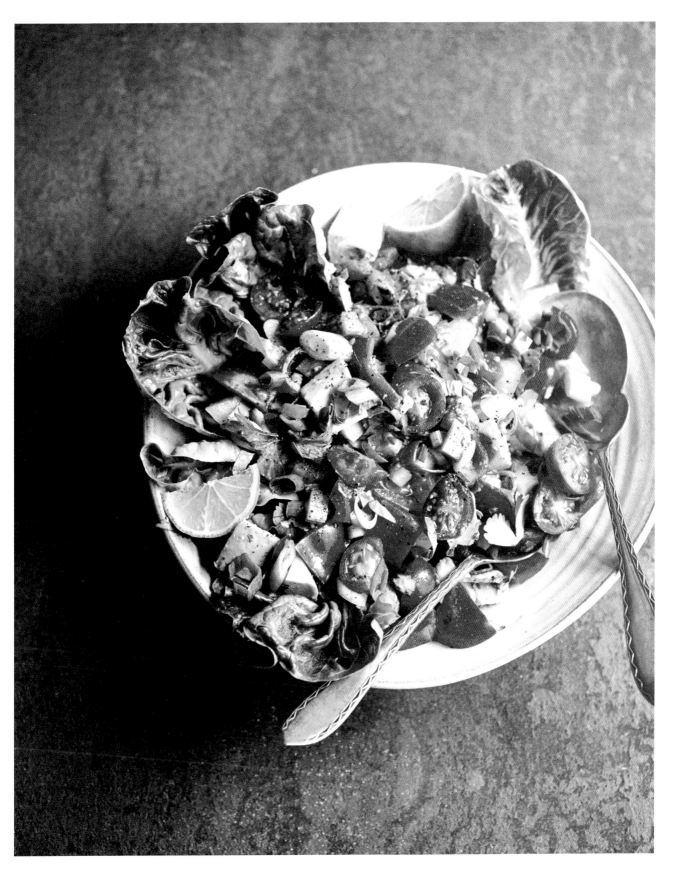

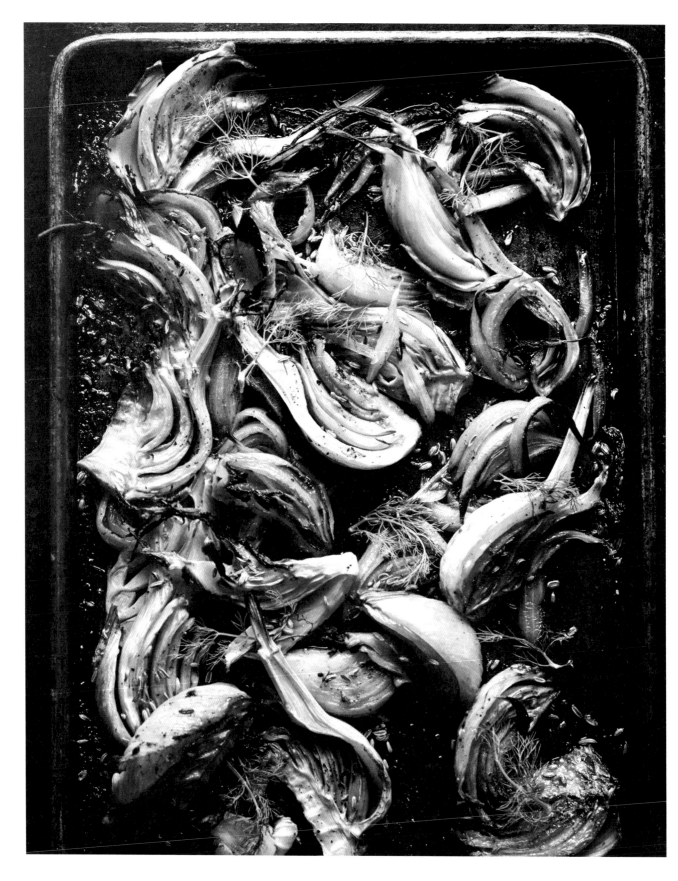

ROAST FENNEL & ONIONS

L

SERVES 6

2 large fennel bulbs (approx. 700g/1lb 9oz), plus fronds to garnish (optional)

2 onions, cut into slim wedges

5 tablespoons extra virgin olive oil

2 teaspoons fennel seeds

1 teaspoon dried or fresh thyme leaves

2 tablespoons butter

salt and plenty of freshly ground black pepper

Per serving
10.5g net carbs, 6.2g fibre, 2.8g protein, 15.5g fat, 204kcal

Fennel can be divisive but we love its aniseedy overtones, especially when combined with the gentle spice of fennel seeds. It's wonderful with roast pork, sausages, fish or poached eggs.

Remove the base of each bulb of fennel and cut away any brown or soft parts of the outer leaves, peeling away as little as possible. Cut each bulb in half from stalk to base, then cut each half into 5 or 6 wedges. Put the fennel into a saucepan of boiling, salted water and cook for 10 minutes.

Preheat the oven to 220°C/200°C fan/425°F/gas mark 7.

When the fennel is ready, drain in a colander and then spread out in a large roasting dish. Add the onion wedges, pour over the oil, then scatter over some seasoning, the fennel seeds and thyme and fleck over the butter.

Roast in the oven for about 20 minutes or until golden brown. Serve straight away scattered with the fennel fronds, if you like, or keep warm until you are ready to serve. Any leftovers can be kept in the fridge for 3 days and reheated in a low oven or in the microwave.

SUPER SLAW

L

SERVES 4

For the salad

3 spring onions, finely chopped

200g (7oz) white or red cabbage, or sprouts, finely shredded

1 apple or 100g (3½oz) cooked beetroot, quartered and grated, or 100g (3½oz) pomegranate seeds

2 celery sticks with leaves, finely sliced

1 small carrot, coarsely grated

½–1 hot green chilli, finely chopped, to taste (optional)

a small bunch (approx. 15g/½oz) of dill, coriander or flat-leaf parsley, stalks finely chopped, leaves torn

For the mustard dressing

2 tablespoons cider vinegar or lemon juice

2 teaspoons Dijon mustard

4 tablespoons extra virgin olive oil

salt and freshly ground black pepper

For the creamy mayo dressing

2 tablespoons mayonnaise

2 tablespoons Greek yogurt or crème fraîche

Per serving
with the mustard dressing
9.9g net carbs, 3.3g fibre,
1.6g protein, 14g fat, 174kcal

with the creamy dressing
11g net carbs, 3.2g fibre,
3.9g protein, 24g fat, 279kcal

To make this slaw, simply shred any member or a mixture of the cabbage family, including Brussels sprouts, to make up the volume. Variety is key to getting a diverse range of nutrients in your diet, so the more colourful the better. If you have a food processor this takes very little time, but you can also use a mandoline or sharp knife. I have collected gadgets over the years and love my Vietnamese carrot shredder and my mother's old cheese slicer; both give quick and interesting cuts to salad vegetables.

We sometimes add a chopped green chilli for a kick of heat or throw in chopped herbs for variation. And, depending on what we are eating with the slaw, we choose a simple clear dressing or a creamy version. In this recipe I've given suggestions for a sweet element: an apple, beetroot or pomegranate seeds. If you would like more protein, add 100g (3½oz) nuts or the Spicy seed crunch on page 150.

Soak the onions for 15 minutes in cold water to dilute their strength.

Combine the mustard dressing ingredients together in a large mixing bowl. If you want to make the creamy mayo dressing, just add the mayonnaise and yogurt to these too. Season to taste, add all the salad ingredients and stir through to combine. Serve straight away or chill for up to 4 hours before serving.

SAUTÉED GREENS WITH CHILLI & GARLIC

U
SERVES 2

2 tablespoons extra virgin olive oil

2 garlic cloves, peeled and lightly crushed with the flat of a knife

½–1 red chilli, depending on heat, finely sliced

200g (7oz) cooked spinach, curly kale, cavolo nero, spring greens or Swiss chard

a squeeze of lemon juice (optional)

salt and freshly ground black pepper

Per serving
1g net carbs, 2.8g fibre,
3.3g protein, 14g fat, 147kcal

I have a theory that people who hate greens just haven't had them cooked by Italians! Tender cooked green leaves dressed in a slick of spicy extra virgin olive oil and garlic is our comfort food and a bowlful will be fought over at the kitchen table. Traditionally, Italians and their Mediterranean neighbours collected wild greens such as chicory, wild rocket, ground elder, cress, nettle and dandelion leaves from the fields, adding fibre and a diversity of vitamins and minerals to their diet. It is a good idea to vary your greens throughout the year, following the seasons and what is available. And by eating greens with olive oil, you help to the release the valuable fat-soluble vitamins.

How to prepare spinach: Baby spinach can be added straight to the pan and doesn't need pre-boiling. Older, tougher spinach leaves need to be picked from their fibrous white stems, which can be discarded. Wash the leaves and steam in the residual water for 5 minutes until tender. Drain well. 300g (10½oz) raw leaves is enough to make 200g (7oz) boiled and squeezed leaves. Frozen whole-leaf spinach is ideal to use; a 900g (2lb) bag will give you about 400g (14oz) after defrosting and squeezing.

How to prepare curly kale, cavolo nero (black kale) or spring greens: Pinch the rib around the middle of the leaf and pull the leaves away by running your fingers up and down the hard stalk. Discard the stalks. Wash the leaves under cold running water. Roughly shred the leaves and cook them in salted boiling water for up to 10 minutes until tender. Drain, and squeeze out the water when cool to the touch. The weight doesn't change after boiling so 200g (7oz) raw leaves is enough to make 200g (7oz) boiled leaves.

How to prepare Swiss chard: My Italian mother-in-law would never have thrown away the stems, but they do have a strong minerally flavour, so they are not to everyone's taste. They have to be cooked separately to the leaves unless chopped very finely, as they take longer to cook. Cut away the thick white or rainbow-coloured stems from just under the leaf. Discard the stems or cut them finely and boil them in salted water for 10–15 minutes until tender. Boil the leaves for about 5 minutes until tender. Drain well. 300g (10½oz) is enough to make 200g (7oz) boiled leaves.

Variation
Use half olive oil and half toasted sesame oil and add in a thumb-sized piece of finely chopped ginger with the garlic.

Heat the oil in a large frying pan and, when hot, add the garlic, chilli, salt and pepper. Fry for a couple of minutes until they soften but watch they don't burn. Add the cooked and drained leaves and fry for about 5 minutes, stirring constantly. If using baby spinach, cook this from raw in batches in the pan. Add a squeeze of lemon juice, if you like.

RAINBOW STIR-FRY

U

SERVES 4

1 courgette

1 red pepper

1 small leek

2 tablespoons extra virgin olive oil

1 fat garlic clove, peeled and lightly
    crushed with the flat side of a knife

a small bunch of thyme leaves or
    1 sprig of rosemary or 1 teaspoon
    dried thyme

salt and freshly ground black pepper

Per serving
3.9g net carbs, 1.3g fibre,
1.2g protein, 7g fat, 86kcal

This very simple but very effective idea came from a visit to the wonderful restaurant Tweedies in Paphos. The chef, Craig, made a first course with stir-fried vegetables and prawns. I loved the way he peeled and shaved everyday vegetables and turned them into this gorgeous bowl of colour and flavour. This is my version turned into a side dish that goes with everything from meat and fish to eggs or fried tofu.

Peel the courgette into ribbons with a vegetable peeler. Cut the red pepper into thin strips. Cut the leek into 2–3 lengths and then slice it lengthways into shreds. Wash it in cold water to get rid of any mud.

Heat the oil in a large frying pan or wok and fry the garlic clove and thyme for about 1 minute. Add the vegetables and seasoning and stir-fry for about 5 minutes until wilted. Serve straight away.

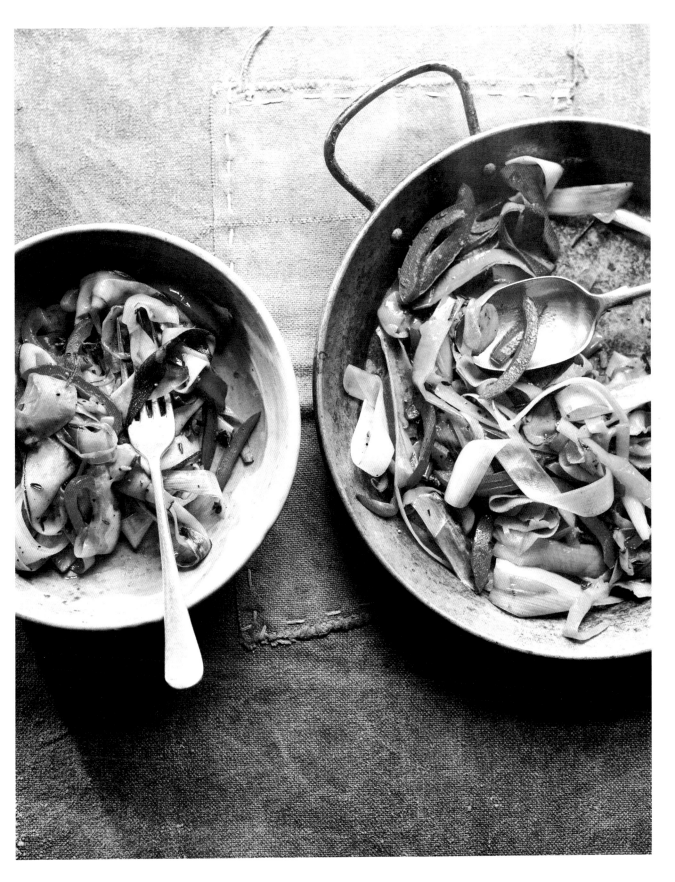

FLAVIO'S OVEN-BAKED SPICY CHIPS

L
SERVES 4

600g (1lb 5oz) celeriac, swede, okra
or sweet potato, or a mixture
2 tablespoons extra virgin olive oil
salt

For the spicy chips
1 tablespoon smoked paprika
1 teaspoon cayenne pepper
2 teaspoons garlic powder

Per serving
of celeriac chips
11.1g net carbs, 2.7g fibre,
2.3g protein, 7.2g fat, 122kcal

of swede chips
3.5g net carbs, 0g fibre,
0.5g protein, 6.9g fat, 76kcal

of okra chips
6.4g net carbs, 4.8g fibre,
2.9g protein, 7g fat, 109kcal

of sweet potato chips
25.7g net carbs, 4.5g fibre,
2.4g protein, 6.8g fat, 188kcal

This recipe was really popular in *The Reverse Your Diabetes Cookbook*, so I have included it here, too. Since potatoes are out on a low-carb diet, we've come up with some even-better-than-the-spud alternatives packed with colour and flavour by using okra or roots such as swede and celeriac. Try one on its own or a mixture together. A word of warning however: none of these vegetables contain the starch that potato does so they won't be as crispy, but they will have more flavour. To cook crispy celeriac chips, Jenny uses her air-fryer, which is speedy and effective.

Preheat the oven to 220°C/200°C fan/425°F/gas mark 7. Line 1–2 baking trays with baking parchment.

Peel the root vegetables and cut into even-sized chips. Rinse the okra and dry with kitchen paper. Don't mix the okra with the other vegetables as they have a different cooking time.

Toss the root veg chips or okra in a bowl with the oil and salt and make sure they are evenly coated. For the spicy chips, make up the spice mixture and add with the oil and salt in the bowl. Place the chips into the prepared tray/s and cook the okra for about 15 minutes and the root veg chips for 20–25 minutes or until golden brown and crispy.

Serve straight away.

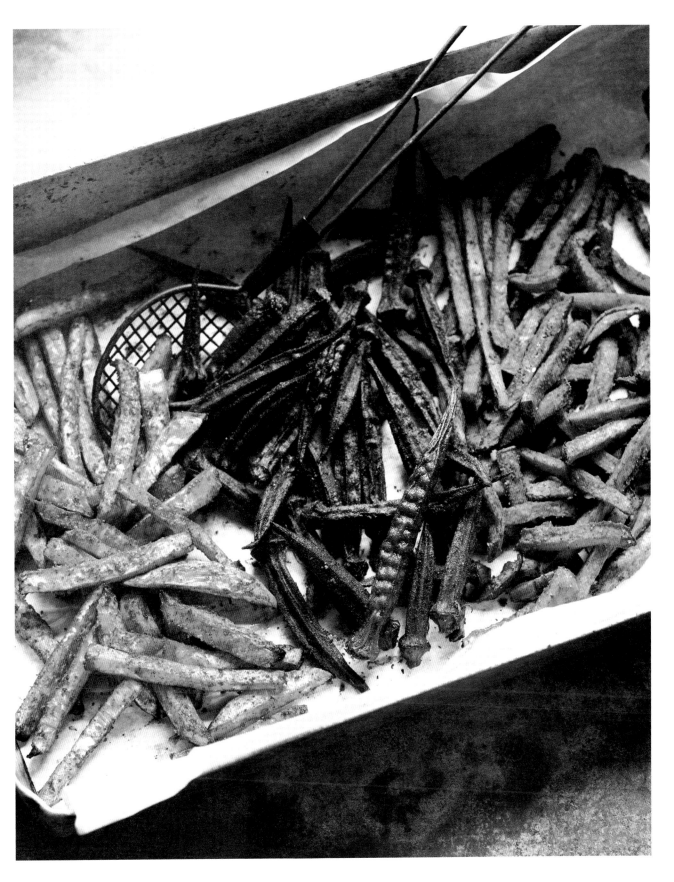

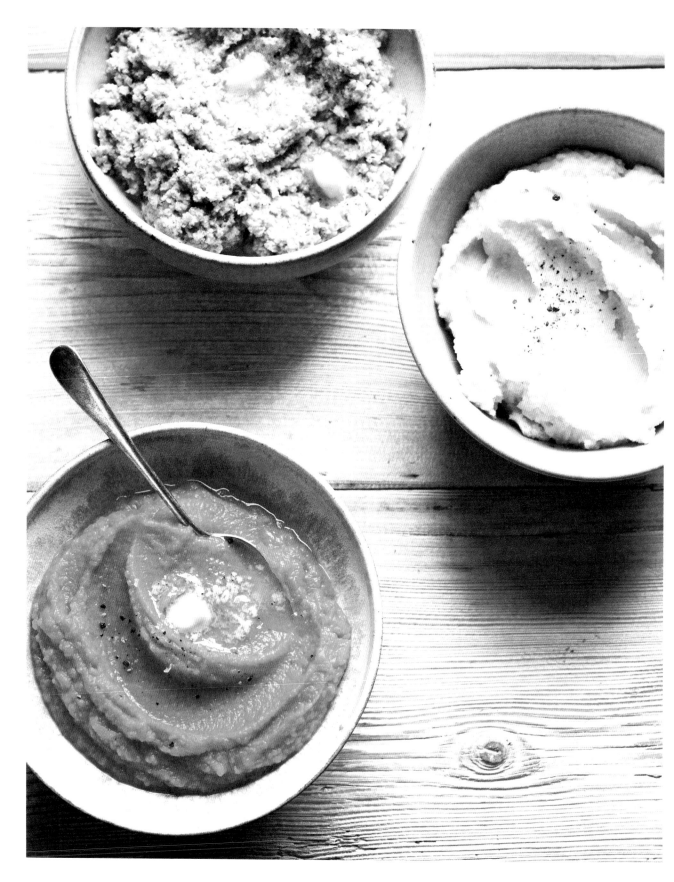

LOW-CARB MASH

U

SERVES 4

400g (14oz) low-carb vegetable(s), such as celeriac, pumpkin, swede, Brussels sprouts, cauliflower or broccoli or, or a mixture

25g (1oz) butter or extra virgin olive oil, plus extra to serve

25–75ml (1–2½fl oz) cow's milk, almond milk, cream or crème fraîche, as necessary

½ teaspoon ground nutmeg (optional)

salt and freshly ground black pepper

Per serving
of sprout mash
5.4g net carbs, 3.8g fibre,
3.6g protein, 5.6g fat, 91kcal

of cauli mash
3.3g net carbs, 2g fibre,
2.2g protein, 5.6g fat, 73kcal

of swede mash
2.6g net carbs, 0g fibre,
0.6g protein, 5.6g fat, 60kcal

of pumpkin mash
6.3g net carbs, 0.5g fibre,
1.3g protein, 5.6g fat, 74kcal

of celeriac mash
7.7g net carbs, 1.8g fibre,
1.8g protein, 5.6g fat, 90kcal

Here are a few ideas for low-carb mash. Potatoes, sweet potatoes and butternut squash are off the menu if you are keeping your carbs low, but pumpkin, cauliflower and some root vegetables, such as celeriac and swede, are perfect for making delicious mash with a fraction of the carbs of the potato version. Celeriac mash, for example, contains under 8g carbs per serving compared to potato mash at 24g. You can use your potato masher but, as many of the root vegetables are fibrous, a food processor or stick blender gives a better creamy texture. Any leftovers keep well in the fridge for up to 4 days and can be reheated easily.

By using the leaves and stalk of the cauliflower you get a lot more mash. Cut the stalks into smaller pieces than the rest of the vegetable and cook first. Add the leaves last to ensure even cooking.

As some veg are more absorbent than others, you may have to alter the amount of milk you use. To reduce the carbs further, use almond milk or cream instead of cow's milk.

Peel and dice the celeriac, pumpkin and/or swede into about 2cm (¾in) cubes; cut the ends off the sprouts and peel off any dirty leaves. Cut the cauliflower and broccoli into small florets and chop the stalks into 1cm (½in) dice. Steam or boil the vegetables until just tender. Drain well.

Blend the cooked veg with the remaining ingredients in a food processor or with a stick blender until you have a soft, smooth mash. Taste and adjust the seasoning as necessary. Spoon into a warm bowl and dot with butter to serve.

ITALIAN ROAST VEGETABLES

L

SERVES 4

5 tablespoons extra virgin olive oil

1 aubergine, cut into 1cm (½in) slices

1 courgette, cut into 1cm (½in) slices

1 red or yellow pepper, cut into finger-width strips

1 onion, cut into finger-width wedges

2 sprigs of rosemary, thyme or sage

2 garlic cloves, unpeeled and lightly crushed

a large pinch of salt and freshly ground black pepper

Per serving
6.4g net carbs, 3.4g fibre,
1.6g protein, 16g fat, 185kcal

This is our staple recipe for roasting vegetables Italian style. Always tuck the herbs under the vegetables to give flavour and stop them burning and space the vegetables out so that they all roast rather than steam in a pile. These are great as an accompaniment to meat, fish and poached eggs, as a base for pasta sauces, or try them with a soft, creamy burrata or buffalo mozzarella and a scattering of basil.

Preheat the oven to 220°C/200°C fan/425°F/gas mark 7 and grease a baking tray with a little of the oil.

Put the vegetables into a bowl with the olive oil and seasoning and toss to combine. Spread them evenly over the tray in one layer (you may have to use 2 trays). Tuck the herbs underneath the vegetables and add the garlic. Roast for 25–30 minutes until cooked through and golden brown on top.

ROAST AUBERGINE & BUTTERNUT SQUASH

L

SERVES 2

250g (9oz) butternut squash, unpeeled, cut into 1cm (½in) wedges

1 onion, sliced into wedges

1 small aubergine (approx. 250g/9oz), cut into 1.5cm (⅝in) slices

3 tablespoons extra virgin olive oil

1 tablespoon toasted sesame seeds (optional)

salt and freshly ground black pepper

Although higher in carbs than most of our vegetables of choice, butternut squash is great in a Rainbowl (page 150) with shredded kale, soft-boiled eggs, fish, Spicy seed crunch (page 150), cooked chicken or a green salad.

Preheat the oven to 240°C/220°C fan/475°F/gas mark 9 and line a baking tray with baking parchment.

Spread the vegetables out over the prepared baking tray and brush over the oil. Evenly scatter over the seeds and some seasoning and roast for 20 minutes or until the vegetables are tender and lightly browned. Serve hot or at room temperature.

Per serving
21.4g net carbs, 8.5g fibre, 3.5g protein, 22.7g fat, 316kcal

BAKED "BEANS"

U

SERVES 6

200g (7oz) smoked bacon lardons

75g (2¾oz) carrot, finely chopped

2 celery sticks, finely chopped

1 onion, finely chopped

2 tablespoons extra virgin olive oil

350g (12oz) cauliflower, chopped
   into small pieces roughly the size
   of a marble

½ teaspoon smoked paprika

2 teaspoons English or Dijon mustard

1 tablespoon red or white wine or
   cider vinegar

2 tablespoons tomato purée

400g (14oz) can of chopped tomatoes

400ml (14fl oz) vegetable or
   chicken stock

salt and freshly ground black pepper

Per serving
3.5g net carbs, 3.4g fibre,
4.4g protein, 7g fat, 101kcal

One of my earliest cooking memories is standing on a chair in the kitchen stirring curry powder into a saucepan of baked beans – everyone has to start somewhere! Many years later, I spent ages recreating baked beans following an old Southern American recipe: smoking my own pork belly then using that with dried beans and cooking them together really slowly, cowboy style. They were delicious but laden with sugar and starchy carbs. So, this is my third go at making baked beans; this time there are no beans but all the comforting flavour, colour and texture of the traditional version to pile on my plate. This is perfect with a cooked breakfast, sausages, eggs, topped with grated Cheddar on Hot buttered toast (page 51) or on the Chaffles on page 44.

Fry the lardons, carrot, celery and onion with seasoning in the olive oil in a large saucepan over a medium heat for 12–15 minutes or until the vegetables have softened. Add the cauliflower and paprika and stir everything through to coat in the oil in the pan.

Now add the remaining ingredients and bring to the boil, then reduce the heat and simmer for 30 minutes or until the cauliflower is easily crushed by a wooden spoon against the side of the pan. Taste and adjust the flavour as you like with seasoning, spices or even a little curry powder!

BRUSSELS SPROUT, BACON & LEEK HASH

L

SERVES 4

1 medium leek, roughly chopped

6 rashers of smoked streaky
  bacon, cut into strips, or
  100g (3½oz) bacon lardons

1 tablespoon extra virgin olive oil

25g (1oz) butter

500g (1lb 2oz) Brussels sprouts

salt and freshly ground black pepper

Per serving
of hash
6g net carbs, 5.7g fibre,
18g protein, 20g fat, 285kcal

of hash and 2 eggs
8.8g net carbs, 5.7g fibre,
32g protein, 29g fat, 428kcal

"Sprouts are not just for Christmas" is my motto. This wonderful combination works alongside a myriad of main courses, such as sausages, or the Swedish meatballs on page 124. With the addition of eggs it becomes a meal in its own right. The hash keeps well in the fridge and can be reheated quickly in the microwave or in a covered pan over a low heat.

Fry the leek and bacon in the oil and butter (with a little seasoning if you are using lardons) in a large frying pan or wok over a medium heat for about 10 minutes. Stir frequently and shake the pan to distribute the leeks and bacon evenly.

Cut the ends (bases) off the sprouts. Pull off any grubby leaves and cut them in half. Put the sprouts into boiling salted water for 5 minutes or until just cooked but still green.

When the leeks are soft and becoming transparent, drain the sprouts and add them to the pan. Stir everything together and season to taste.

Variation

To cook the hash with eggs, remove half the mixture from the pan and set aside, as you have to do this in 2 batches. Make 4 indentations in the cooked hash and crack an egg into each one. Scatter over a little seasoning and put on the lid. Continue to cook over a low–medium heat until the eggs are done to your liking.

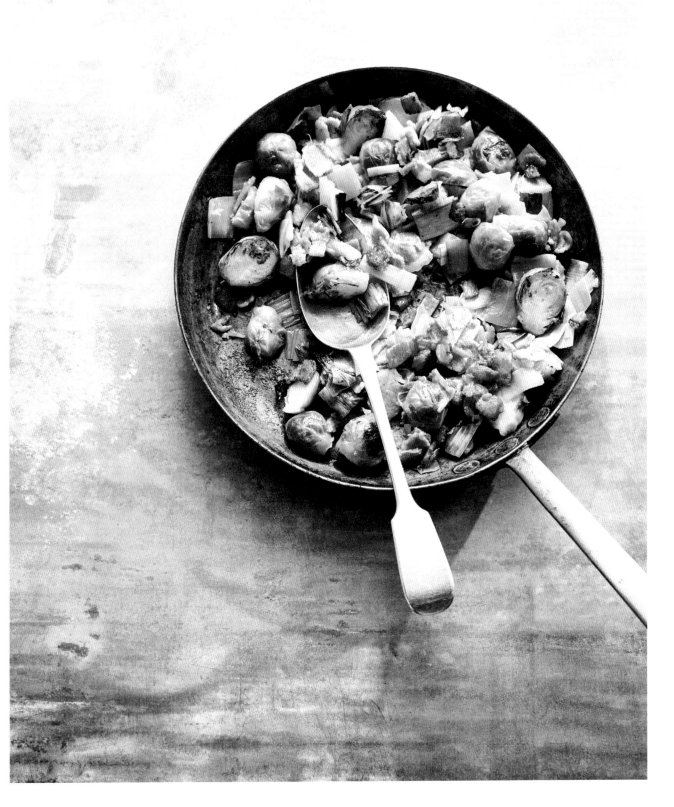

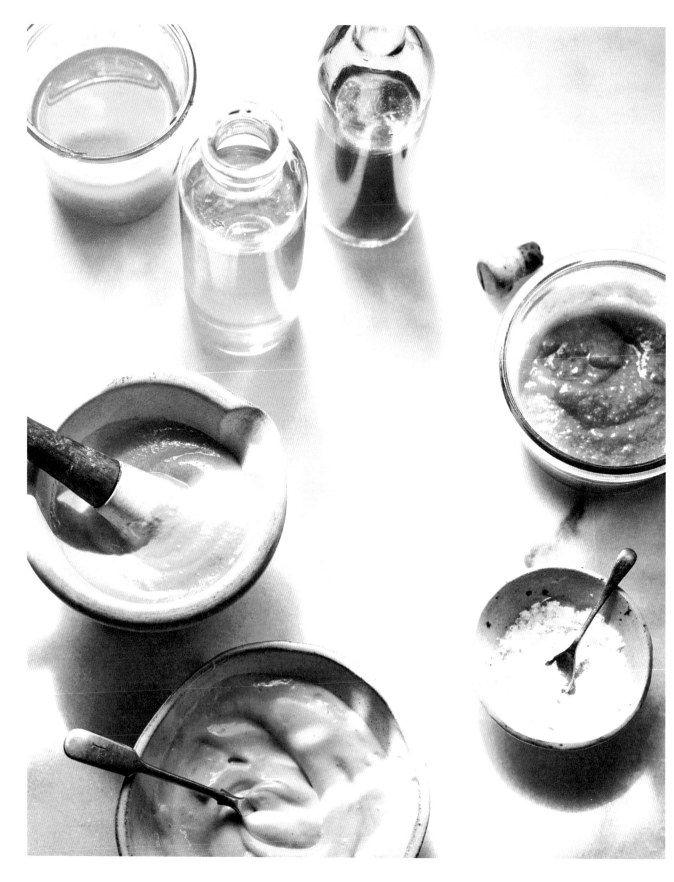

OUR FAVOURITE SALAD DRESSINGS

I'm convinced more people would enjoy salad if it was served with a good dressing, so here are some of our favourite recipes for dressing a bowl of the green stuff. And remember, by eating greens with fats you are making the fat-soluble vitamins more accessible. For more dressing ideas and inspiration, have a look at our book *Around the World in Salads*.

ONE-MINUTE MAYONNAISE

Take your pick which oil to use from the list below but don't be tempted to use extra virgin olive oil in this mayo, as it is too strong and bitter. This is the basic recipe, but you can flavour it with a little grated fresh or mashed roasted garlic, lemon zest, chopped chives, chipotle or curry powder.

SERVES 4

1 medium egg

1 heaped teaspoon Dijon mustard

1 teaspoon lemon juice

150ml (5fl oz) cold-pressed avocado or rapeseed oil

½ teaspoon salt

a few twists of freshly ground black pepper

Put all the ingredients into the narrow, tall mixing bowl of a stick blender. If you don't have one, use a narrow, tall jam jar instead. There should only be up to 1cm (½in) of room around the stick blender.

Put the stick blender to the bottom and whizz for 30 seconds or until you see a thick mayonnaise forming. Slowly lift the blender upwards to mix all the oil in. If there is a little on top, you can stir this in.

Now taste the mayo; at this point you can stir in more lemon juice, mustard, seasoning or other flavourings. It will keep for up to 3 days in the fridge.

Per serving made with any of the oils above
0.5g net carbs, 0g fibre, 2g protein, 36g fat, 334kcal

GARLIC MAYONNAISE

This is ideal to make to serve alongside the Chicken souvlaki on page 112. Simply add ½–1 teaspoon of grated garlic to the One-minute mayonnaise to taste.

Per serving
0.5g net carbs, 0.5g fibre, 2g protein, 36g fat, 335kcal

VEGAN AQUAFABA MAYONNAISE

Aquafaba is the water from canned chickpeas or other beans and can be used in recipes instead of egg white. It should be fairly thick, so reduce it by half over a medium heat when it is straight out of the can. Cool and use as below or for cakes and meringues.

SERVES 8

4 tablespoons (60ml) thick aquafaba (if not thick, see above)

1 tablespoon vegan cider vinegar

1 tablespoon lemon juice

1 heaped teaspoon mustard powder or vegan Dijon mustard

a good pinch of salt

300ml (10fl oz) cold-pressed rapeseed or avocado oil

Put the aquafaba, vinegar, lemon juice, mustard and salt into the base of a stick blender or tall food processor. Start blending the ingredients together while slowly pouring a thin stream of the oil into the blender while it is running. It will thicken and make a mayonnaise. Do not over-blend; as soon as it is thick and you have used all the oil, stop. Season to taste and keep cool. The mayonnaise can be put into a jar and kept in the fridge for up to 5 days.

Per serving made with any of the oils above
0.5g net carbs, 0g fibre, 0g protein, 35g fat, 315kcal

CLASSIC VINAIGRETTE

My earliest memory of cooking is shaking the vinaigrette in a jar for my mum as she prepared salad for us all. She would get me to taste it and decide if it needed more of any of the ingredients. In that simple task, she gave me confidence in my taste. Thanks, Mum.

SERVES 8

2 tablespoons red wine vinegar

8 tablespoons extra virgin olive oil

½ teaspoon salt

a good pinch of freshly ground black pepper

1 heaped teaspoon Dijon mustard

1 tablespoon lemon juice

1 small garlic clove, grated

½ teaspoon honey (optional)

Put all the ingredients in a jar and shake until emulsified. Keep any remaining dressing in the jar in the fridge for up to a week.

Per serving
0.5g net carbs, 0g fibre, 0g protein, 13g fat, 118kcal

MISO DRESSING

Our boys love the umami hit of miso, the fermented soybean paste. We use it on the Miso salmon recipe on page 138 and you can make it into soup or stir it into soups and sauces, but here it combines with tahini, the sesame seed paste, to give a tangy, creamy dressing ideal for salads and slaws.

SERVES 4

2 tablespoons white miso paste

1 teaspoon finely grated fresh ginger

2 tablespoons extra virgin olive oil

2 tablespoons mirin or 2 teaspoons honey

½–1 teaspoon lemon juice (optional)

½ teaspoon toasted sesame oil

Whisk the ingredients together in a bowl with 1 tablespoon of water, whisking in a little at a time to dilute the sauce to a pouring consistency. This dressing will keep for up to a week, covered, in the fridge.

Per serving
7.6g net carbs, 0.3g fibre, 0.6g protein, 9.1g fat, 119kcal

GOLDEN TAHINI & TURMERIC DRESSING

This golden combination of tahini (sesame paste) and anti-inflammatory turmeric is not only delicious but beautiful on soft-boiled eggs, roast vegetables, such as the Roast aubergine & butternut squash on page 174, or in the Rainbowl on page 150.

SERVES 4

2 tablespoons tahini

2 tablespoons extra virgin olive oil

1 tablespoon lemon juice

½–1 teaspoon ground turmeric

¼ teaspoon chilli powder, hot smoked paprika or cayenne pepper (optional)

salt and freshly ground black pepper

Mix all the ingredients together in a small bowl or glass jar with 3 tablespoons of water and whisk or shake together to combine. Taste the dressing and add seasoning and more turmeric as you like. Any leftovers will keep for up to a week, covered, in the fridge.

Per serving
1.4g net carbs, 0.7g fibre, 1.3g protein, 10.8g fat, 106kcal

CUCUMBER & TOMATO RAITA

U

SERVES 8

½ small red onion or 5 spring onions,
    finely chopped

175g (6oz) tomatoes (approx.
    1 large or 20 cherry tomatoes),
    finely chopped

½ long cucumber (approx.
    150g/5½oz), finely chopped

300g (10½oz) Greek yogurt

1 heaped tablespoon coriander,
    finely chopped

1 heaped tablespoon mint,
    finely chopped

salt and freshly ground black pepper

Per serving
3.1g net carbs, 0.5g fibre,
2.6g protein, 3.8g fat, 57kcal

I'm used to making cucumber raita but was shown this by Shally Bahtra from Mission Spice for Life cookery school. I love the combination of tomatoes with the cucumber and the fresh herbs. We have these alongside curries or with the Chapattis on page 92.

Soak the red onion in cold water for 10 minutes to dilute its strength.

Drain the onion and mix with the remaining ingredients. Season to taste. Any leftovers will keep, covered, in the fridge for a day or two.

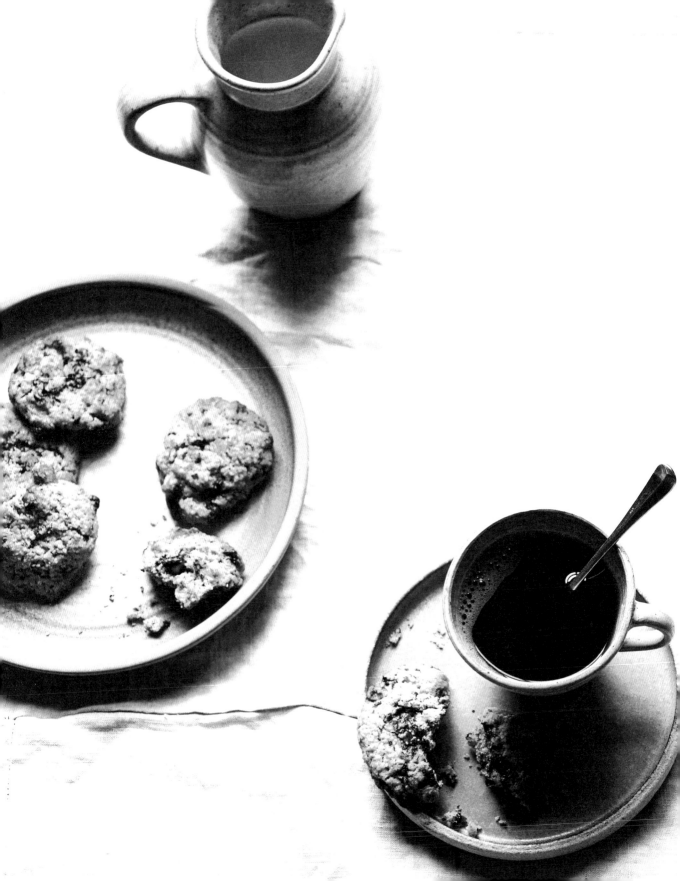

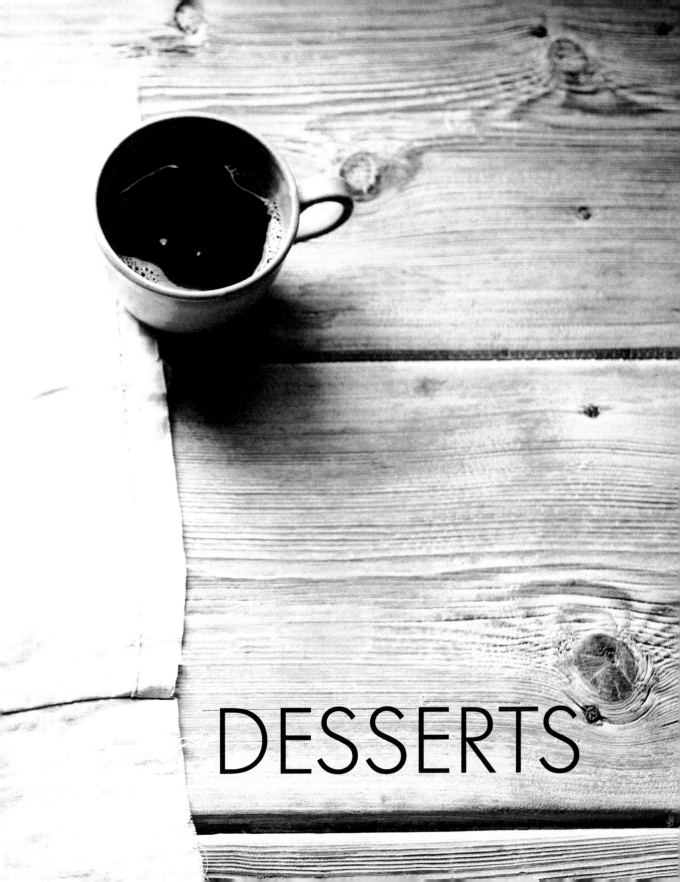

DESSERTS

Jenny, Jen and David would advise you to give desserts a miss as part of a low-carb lifestyle, especially when you are trying to curb your sugar cravings and actively lose weight. However, if you feel you can cope with the occasional treat, as Giancarlo does, here are some decadent desserts for special occasions and petite puddings that are low in carbs and still taste amazing.

In this book we have used some erythritol, a sugar alcohol sweetener that has zero carbs and zero calories. I was opposed to artificial sweeteners for some years but using erythritol does mean you can do so much more than if you're just using the natural sweetness of dates or honey; biscuits have a snap, and you can make meringues and even candy ginger. By using inulin, an insoluble fibre from the root of chicory, you can achieve caramelization similar to burnt sugar; this helps with the flavour and colour of meringues and the crackly crust on a crème brûlée.

Wherever possible we have given you the choice of using minimal dates or honey as a natural sweetener or erythritol. This is because, overall, we want to reduce the sweetness in recipes in whatever form so that you become "low-sugar adapted", as we call it. Even if you use dates or honey, the amounts in the recipes here are so much lower than in commercially made puddings, so you will still be reducing your carb intake. Over time it is likely that your sweet tooth will change, and a shop-bought cake that was once pleasant becomes too sweet.

Which form of sweetener you use depends on how you feel about using artificial sweeteners. You can see the differing values in the nutritional analysis, depending on the sweetener you have used, so you can make informed choices. See www.the goodkitchentable.com for more information on sweeteners and their pros and cons.

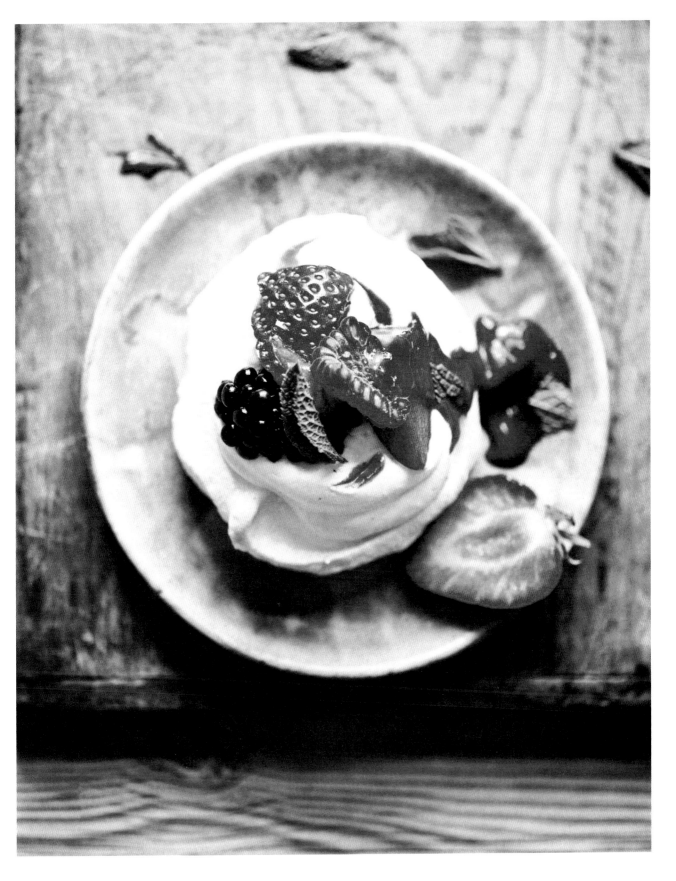

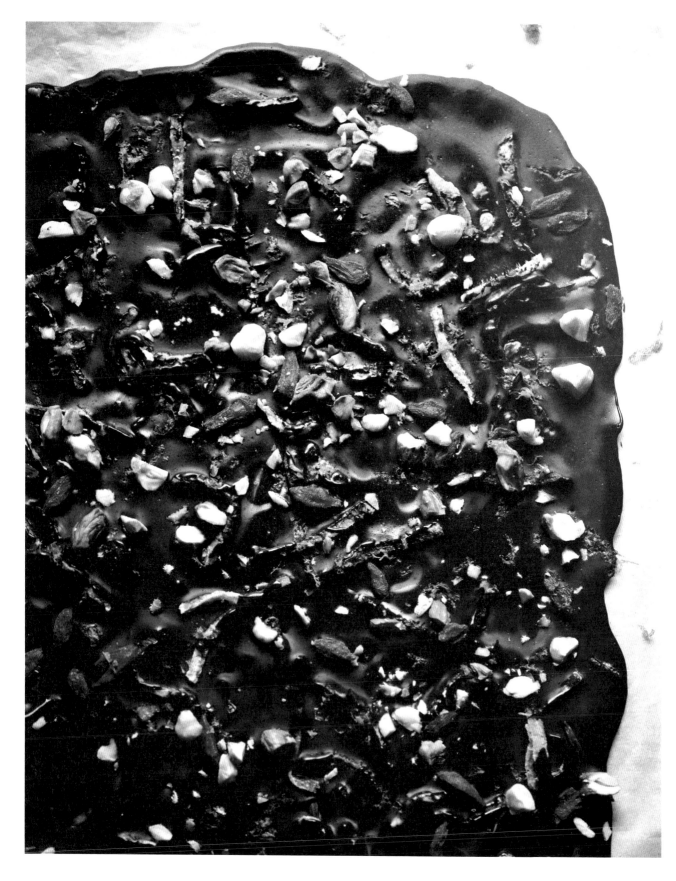

CHOCOLATE GINGER THINS

U
SERVES 8

25g (1oz) fresh ginger, peeled and cut into matchsticks

1 heaped tablespoon erythritol

100g (3½oz) dark chocolate (85% cocoa solids)

15g (½oz) pistachios and/or hazelnuts, roughly chopped, or goji berries, or a mixture of all three

1 teaspoon orange zest (optional)

Per serving
5.2g net carbs, 1.8g fibre, 1.8g protein, 6.6g fat, 82kcal

A shard or two of these is just enough after dinner to satisfy the eternal need for something sweet after a meal. Do keep them out of sight though, as they are devilishly moreish! For a clever temptation-management tip, one of our readers told me that she wraps the portions individually and keeps them in the freezer. She brings out one per day to have after dinner, so that way she isn't tempted to eat them all in one go. This also makes a beautiful edible gift; I wrap the whole slab loosely in baking parchment and tie it up with string.

Put the ginger, 250ml (9fl oz) water and the erythritol into a small saucepan. Bring to the boil and cook over a medium heat for 5–10 minutes until the water evaporates. When it is looking dry, remove the pan from the heat and tip the ginger on to a plate to cool.

Make a bain-marie from a saucepan of hot water with a glass or metal bowl resting over the top. The water should be lower than the bottom of the bowl so that they don't touch.

Start with the bowl off the pan and bring the water to the boil. Remove the pan from the heat and put the bowl over the top of the water. Add the chocolate and wait for it to melt, stirring occasionally. It should only take about 5–10 minutes. Remove the bowl from the pan and leave to cool.

Line a baking tray with baking parchment.

When the chocolate is cool to the touch (about 32°C/90°F) mix in the ginger. Spread the mixture over the prepared tray to a thickness of about 3mm (⅛in). It will be about 17cm (6½in) square. Scatter over the nuts, goji berries and orange zest, if using.

Leave to set in a cool place for about 30 minutes, depending on the temperature of your kitchen. If it is warm, the chocolate can be cooled in the fridge. Once the chocolate has set, break it into shards. At this point it will keep as any bar of chocolate, but as it is thin, it can melt easily so keep in a cool place until you are ready to serve.

BERRIES & WHIPPED CHEESECAKE CREAM

L
SERVES 4

For the cheesecake cream

200g (7oz) Greek yogurt

100ml (3½fl oz) double cream

50g (1¾oz) feta or soft spreadable
goat's cheese or cream cheese

2 teaspoons vanilla extract

4 teaspoons honey or 2 tablespoons
erythritol

For the topping

200g (7oz) frozen or fresh berries,
such as strawberries, raspberries,
blackberries, blueberries,
blackcurrants or redcurrants

a handful of mint tips or edible
flowers (optional)

Per serving
with honey
14.5g net carbs, 1.2g fibre,
5.6g protein, 20.3g fat, 265kcal

with erythritol
8.7g net carbs, 1.2g fibre,
5.5g protein, 20.3g fat, 243kcal

This no-cook dessert can be whisked up at any time of year since you can use frozen or fresh berries. We like to use the berries straight from the freezer as they defrost quickly, and we love the cool crunch as they melt into the cream. The exception are frozen strawberries, which are usually whole and need about 30 minutes to soften.

To get the mildly sour tang of cheesecake that we all love, we have used feta combined with Greek yogurt and cream. You could also use a soft, delicate goat's cheese or cream cheese instead. The vanilla flavour is lovely, but we have also experimented with adding orange or lemon zest and they are gorgeous too.

Whisk all the cheesecake cream ingredients together using an electric or balloon whisk until you have a smooth cream. Spread the cream over a large serving plate. You can dress and eat this straight away or chill until later.

Measure out your frozen or fresh berries and cut any large ones in half. Scatter them over the cheesecake cream and serve straight away. Garnish with the mint leaves or flowers, if using.

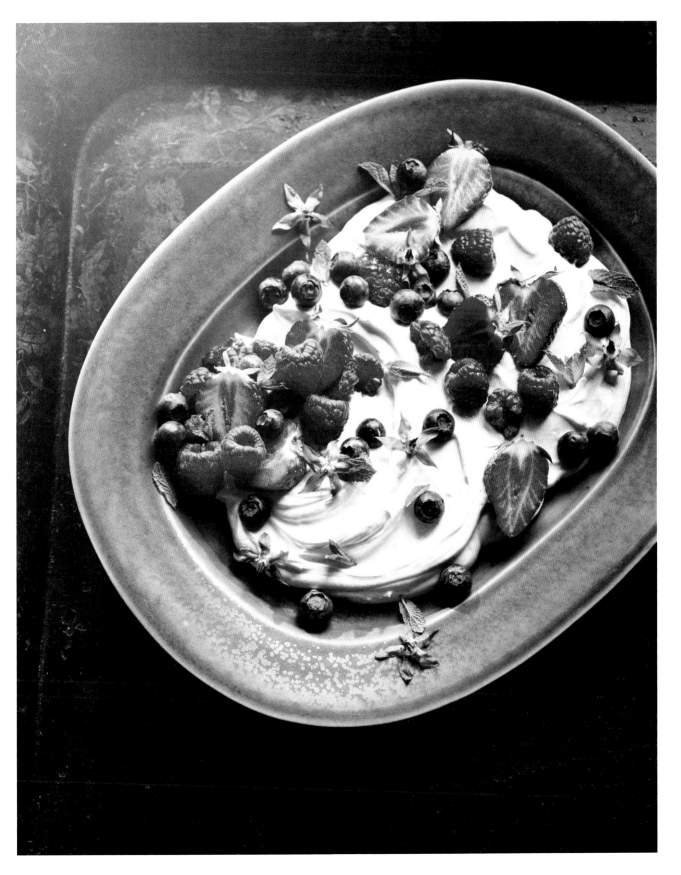

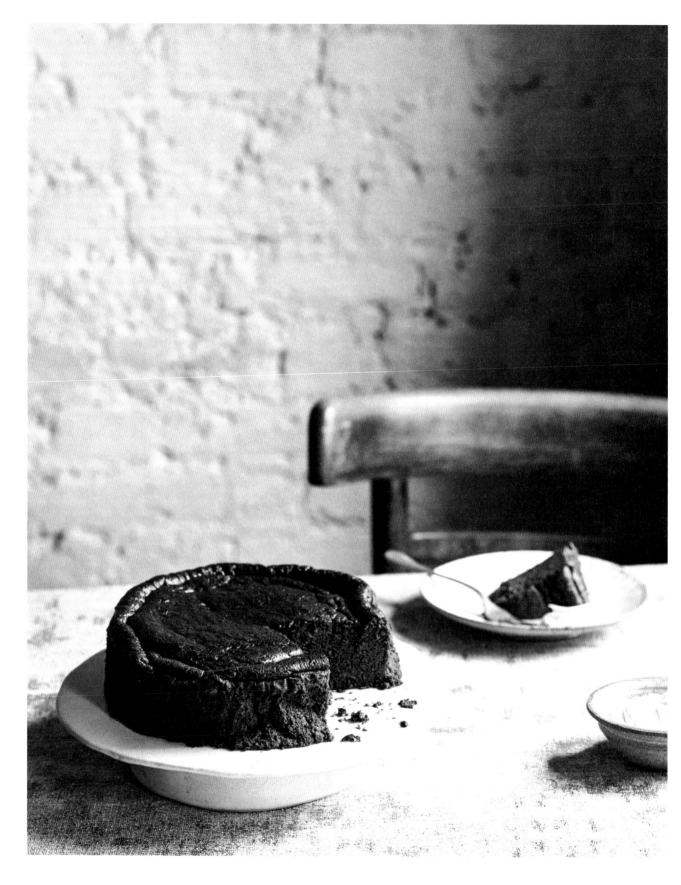

STEFANO'S SQUIDGY CHOCOLATE MOUSSE CAKE

L
SERVES 12

125g (4½oz) butter, plus extra
   for greasing

8 Medjool dates, stoned and roughly
   chopped, or 100g (3½oz) erythritol

100–150ml (3½–5fl oz)
   just-boiled water

200g (7oz) dark chocolate
   (85% cocoa solids or more)

6 eggs

Per serving
with dates
15.1g net carbs, 3.5g fibre,
4.7g protein, 19g fat, 256kcal

with erythritol
4.2g net carbs, 2.4g fibre,
4.4g protein, 19g fat, 212kcal

Warning: this cake is addictive, so enjoy a slice then hide it away or, better still, share it with friends! We were delighted when pâtisserie chef Stefano Borella came up with this nut-free, sugar-free version of a flourless chocolate cake that we had been making for years with sugar. By using minimal dates or erythritol he has achieved the same mousse-like texture and intense chocolate flavour without the sickly-sweet taste of a shop-bought chocolate cake.

Leave it plain, top with whipped cream flavoured with vanilla or serve with Greek yogurt, crème fraîche or soured cream, and berries. If you prefer a slightly wider, shallower cake, you can use a 24cm (9½in) cake tin and cook for 5 minutes less in the oven. It can be eaten in small squares like a brownie with soured cream or Greek yogurt.

Preheat the oven to 190°C/170°C fan/375°F/gas mark 5 and grease a 20cm (8in) high-sided, springform cake tin (see intro if you prefer to make a larger, shallower cake.)

If using the dates, soak them in 150ml (5fl oz) just-boiled water for a few minutes, then mash them to a pulp with a fork or use a stick blender. If using erythritol, dissolve it in 100ml (3½fl oz) just-boiled water in a small saucepan over a medium–high heat. Set aside.

Melt the chocolate and butter together in a bain-marie (a glass or metal bowl over, but not touching, hot water in a saucepan over a medium heat) or in a small bowl in the microwave. Set aside to cool.

Separate the eggs into 2 mixing bowls. Add the date or erythritol mixture to the egg yolks and stir through with a hand whisk or large spoon. Then add the chocolate mixture to the egg yolks and stir again to combine.

Whip the egg whites until just firm enough to stand in peaks. Use a large metal spoon to fold the egg whites into the chocolate mixture. Pour into the prepared cake tin and smooth the surface. Bake for 30–35 minutes. It is ready when the crust feels firm but there should be a slight wobble to it; it will continue setting as it cools. Remove from the oven and leave to cool to room temperature before removing from the tin.

Serve the cake at room temperature or put it into the fridge once cool, where it will keep for a couple of days. The cake is quite fragile so take care transferring it from the tin to a serving plate.

APPLE & CINNAMON PIE

SERVES 8

1 egg yolk, beaten, to glaze

For the pastry

2 Medjool dates or 4 small dates, stoned and finely chopped, or 50g (1¾oz) erythritol

2 tablespoons whole cow's or almond milk or water

200g (7oz) ground almonds

30g (1oz) coconut flour

finely grated zest of ½ lemon

150g (5½oz) cold butter, cut into small cubes

1 egg

2 teaspoons vanilla extract

For the filling

1.2kg (1lb 11oz) eating or cooking apples

2 Medjool dates or 4 small dates, stoned and finely chopped, or 50g (1¾oz) erythritol

4 tablespoons just-boiled water

1 cinnamon stick approx. 8cm (3¼in)

2 teaspoons vanilla extract

3 cloves

We love traditional puddings in our house and with this low-carb, gluten-free pastry we can enjoy one as a treat after a Sunday lunch. You can reduce the carbs a little by substituting some of the apples for blackberries when in season.

Cut 2 pieces of baking parchment about 6cm (2½in) larger than your pie dish, which should measure about 20 x 25cm (8 x 10in).

If using dates for the pastry, put them in a heatproof bowl and pour over the milk, then soften in a microwave. Alternatively, put the dates and milk in a small pan and soften over a medium heat. Use a fork to mash the dates to a purée.

To make the pastry by hand, put the erythritol, if using, almonds, coconut flour and lemon zest into a mixing bowl and add the butter. Use your fingertips to rub the mixture together to form rough pieces. If using dates, use a spoon to push the date mixture through a sieve into a bowl with the almonds, coconut flour and lemon zest, discarding only the thin skins. Add the egg and vanilla and use a fork to mash the ingredients into a well-combined, smooth dough.

If you are using a food processor, simply whizz the pastry ingredients together, adding the erythritol or softened dates as you wish (you don't need to sieve them as the blade will break up the skins).

Scrape the dough out of the food processor or bowl and pile it into a mound in the centre of one of the pieces of baking parchment. Wrap in the parchment and rest in the fridge for at least 20 minutes or for up to a day.

For the filling, peel and core the apples, then slice into 1cm (½in) thick pieces and put into a large saucepan. Put the dates, if using, into the just-boiled water in a small bowl and then mash them with a fork. Add this mixture or the erythritol to the chopped apples with another 4 tablespoons of just-boiled water, the cinnamon, vanilla extract and cloves and cook, covered, for about 10 minutes over a medium heat until the apples have softened. If they become very dry, add another splash of water. Tip the apples into the pie dish and leave to cool to room temperature. If there is a lot of water remaining, pour some away; you should be left with enough to coat the apples but not to be watery.

Per serving
made with dates
24.6g net carbs, 7.3g fibre,
7g protein, 30g fat, 411kcal

made with erythritol
16.4g net carbs, 6.8g fibre,
6.8g protein, 30g fat, 378kcal

Remove the pastry from the fridge and unwrap it. Lay it on to the other piece of baking parchment and put the first piece over the top. Roll out the pastry to about 5mm (¼in) thick and large enough to cover your pie dish. You can check the size by holding the pastry over the dish between the baking parchment.

Preheat the oven to 190°C/170°C fan/375°F/gas mark 5.

Peel off the top sheet of parchment, then turn the pastry and the bottom sheet of parchment on to the pie. Don't worry if the pastry cracks, just push it together and into place. Trim off any excess and use for decorative leaves or freeze for another day.

Brush the top with beaten egg yolk and make a hole in the centre to let the steam out of the pie. Bake for 18–20 minutes or until golden brown.

Serve the pie hot or cold with cream as you like. Leftovers will last for 4 days in the fridge.

ROAST PLUMS WITH ROSEWATER YOGURT

L

SERVES 6

400g (14oz) plums, quartered

6 cardamom pods

15g (½oz) fresh ginger

zest and juice of 1 small orange

1 tablespoon honey or
    2 tablespoons erythritol

10g (¼oz) pistachios, toasted almonds
    or walnuts, roughly chopped

1 tablespoon organic fresh or dried
    rose petals (optional)

For the rosewater yogurt

400g (14oz) Greek yogurt

1 teaspoon finely grated orange zest

2 teaspoons honey or 1 heaped
    tablespoon erythritol

a few drops–¼ teaspoon rosewater

Per serving
with honey
16.7g net carbs, 1.2g fibre,
5g protein, 7.7g fat, 154kcal

with erythritol
11.8g net carbs, 1.2g fibre,
5g protein, 7.7g fat, 136kcal

I love the delicate flavour of rosewater and have collected bottles of it over the years, from the Petals of the Valley brand in Wales, to Bulgaria, which is famous for its valley of the roses, to your average supermarket versions. They all vary in flavour and strength, so it's best to add it drop by drop so you don't overdo it.

I like to serve this dessert in vintage champagne or small wine glasses that I've picked up at car boot sales. Do use peaches or apricots if you can't find plums, or even drained canned apricots.

Preheat the oven to 220°C/200°C fan/425°F/gas mark 7.

Put the plums in an ovenproof dish just larger than the plums, as you don't want too much space around them. Crush the cardamom pods to release the seeds and then crush the seeds in a pestle and mortar or finely chop them with a sharp knife. Scatter them over the plums.

Peel the ginger with a teaspoon – it gets into all the nooks and crannies. Grate it finely into a bowl, then squeeze the juice from the pulp over the plums and discard the fibrous part. Scatter over the orange zest, then pour over the orange juice and 6 tablespoons of water. Drizzle with the honey or scatter over the erythritol.

Roast the plums for 20–30 minutes or until the fruit has softened. This will depend on the ripeness of the fruit. Divide the fruit between 6 glasses and leave to cool to room temperature.

Mix the yogurt with the orange zest and your chosen sweetener and then add the rosewater, a drop at a time, to taste. Top the plums with the yogurt and scatter over the nuts and the rose petals, if using.

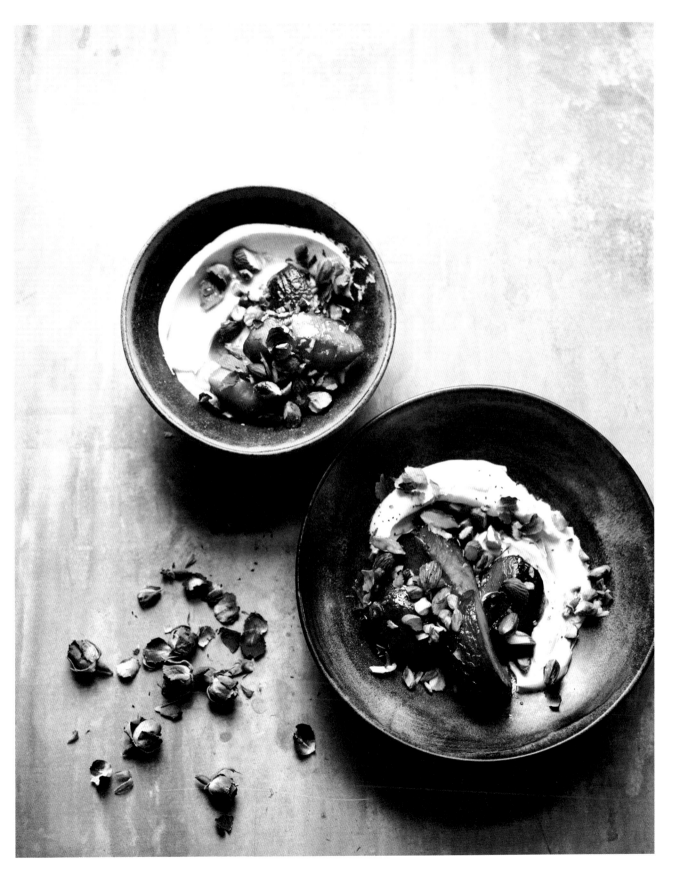

MINI PAVLOVAS

L
SERVES 8

For the meringues

50g (1¾oz) erythritol

50g (1¾oz) inulin powder

3 egg whites (90g/3¼oz)

For the raspberry coulis

200g (7oz) raspberries or
    strawberries, fresh or frozen

1 teaspoon vanilla extract

2 tablespoons erythritol or
    2 teaspoons honey (optional)

For the topping

200ml (7fl oz) whipping cream

2 teaspoons vanilla extract

400g (14oz) fresh berries, such
    as strawberries, raspberries
    and blackberries

8 small mint leaves (optional)

Per serving

6.9g net carbs, 6.8g fibre,
3g protein, 15.8g fat, 191kcal

Our pâtisserie chef, Stefano Borella, loves a challenge. While he was caramelizing the lemon tart using inulin, a powdered insoluble fibre derived from chicory, he wondered about using it combined with the sweetness of erythritol for meringues. It worked brilliantly and now you can eat meringue with a wonderful flavour and still be sugar free. Use fresh eggs for these pavlovas, the more recently laid the better. We use frozen berries in winter and fresh berries in summer to make the coulis. Most of the dessert can be made in advance but the finished pavlova should be assembled just before serving.

Preheat the oven to 110°C/90°C fan/225°F/gas mark ¼. Line a large baking sheet with baking parchment.

Make sure your mixing bowl is thoroughly dry and grease-free. Powder the erythritol in a small food processor so it resembles icing sugar. Mix it in a bowl with the inulin.

Whisk the egg whites in a stand mixer or with an electric whisk until they have formed an opaque foam that forms soft peaks around the sides of the bowl. Add the erythritol and inulin mixture a tablespoon at a time. Keep whisking until you have a stiff, glossy foam. Use a large metal spoon to shape meringues about 6–8cm (2½–3¼in) wide and about 5cm (2in) apart on the prepared baking sheet – they should be about 3cm (1¼in) high – and use the spoon to create a dip in the centre for the cream. You can also do this with a piping bag.

Bake the meringues for 45–50 minutes or until set but still flexible and lightly browned. The meringues can now be left inside the oven to dry them out or you can remove them from the oven and let the meringues come to room temperature. When the meringues are bone dry, they are best left out, not in a container, and will keep for 4 days. It is best not to dress the meringues with cream until you are ready to eat them, or they will soften.

Meanwhile, make the coulis by blending the raspberries with the vanilla and, depending on the natural sweetness of the berries, the erythritol or honey. If the pips bother you, sieve the coulis. Transfer to a serving jug and set aside. This will keep in the fridge for up to 3 days. Stir before use.

Whip the cream with the vanilla to form soft peaks; don't overwhip it though or you will get butter. Hull fresh strawberries and halve or quarter any large berries. Keep the berries in the fridge for up to 3 hours. Just before serving, spoon the cream over the meringues and top with the fruits and a scattering of mint leaves, if using. Serve with the coulis on the side.

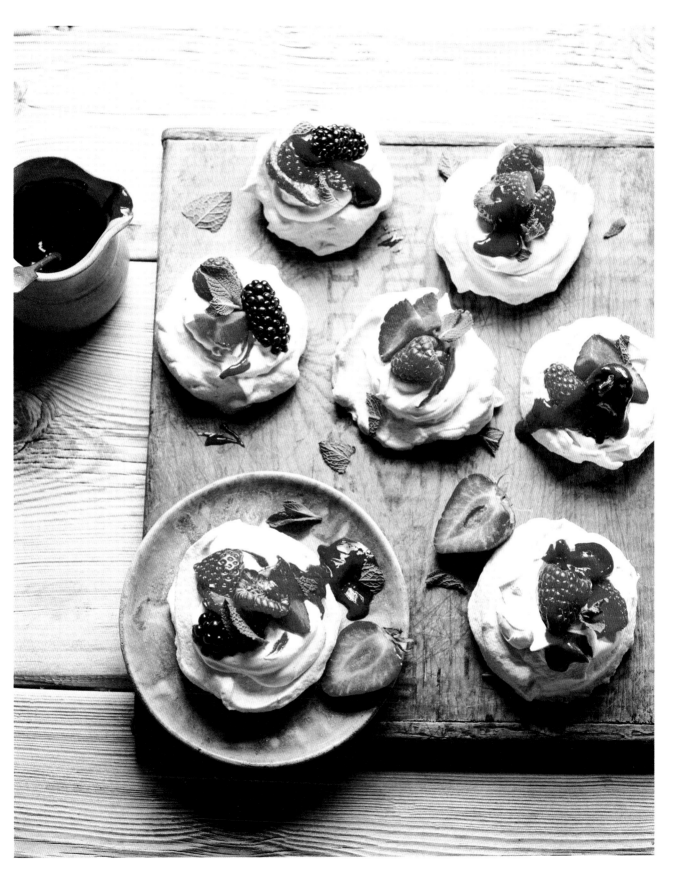

HAZELNUT & CHOCOLATE COOKIES

L

SERVES 12

50g (1¾oz) whole blanched hazelnuts

50g (1¾oz) ground almonds

25g (1oz) butter

20g (¾oz) erythritol

10g (¼oz) stevia

½ teaspoon baking powder

1 egg

2 teaspoons vanilla extract

20g (¾oz) dark chocolate (85% cocoa solids), roughly chopped

Per cookie
1.3g net carbs, 0.9g fibre,
2.2g protein, 7.5g fat, 80kcal

Forgive the two sugar replacements but after many trials using natural sweeteners as well as artificial ones, we worked out that this combination gives a pleasant sweetness without an obvious aftertaste and the perfect crunch to the cookies. (Dates and honey made the cookies soft.) We have used small quantities of stevia, which can taste bitter, but when combined with erythritol it gives a pleasant, sweet taste and mitigates the cooling sensation of erythritol. (See the photo on page 182.)

Preheat the oven to 190°C/170°C fan/375°F/gas mark 5 and line a baking tray with baking parchment.

Scatter the hazelnuts over the prepared tray and toast for 8–10 minutes or until golden brown. Use the parchment to pour them on to a large plate to cool. Return the parchment to the tray and set aside.

Use a sharp knife or a food processor to roughly chop the cooled hazelnuts and pour into a mixing bowl. Add the remaining ingredients and stir together with a large metal spoon until well combined.

Use a dessertspoon to spoon 12 heaped mounds on to the lined tray, spaced about 4cm (1½in) apart.

Bake the cookies for 10 minutes or until lightly golden. Remove from the oven and leave to cool on a wire rack before serving. They can be stored in an airtight container for up to a week or frozen for up to 3 months.

LUSCIOUS LEMON TART

L
SERVES 12

For the sweet pastry

30g (1oz) unsalted butter, plus extra for greasing

175g (6oz) ground almonds

1 teaspoon xanthan gum

2 teaspoons vanilla extract

2 teaspoons honey or 2 tablespoons erythritol

1 large egg

For the filling

finely grated zest and juice of 2 lemons

3 large eggs

75g (2¾oz) honey or 100g (3½oz) erythritol

200ml (7fl oz) double cream

For the glaze

1 tablespoon powdered inulin (optional)

Per serving
with honey
8.5g net carbs, 2.1g fibre, 5.3g protein, 20g fat, 240kcal

with erythritol
2.4g net carbs, 2.1g fibre, 5.3g protein, 20g fat, 218kcal

This beautiful lemon tart has all the typical bittersweet tang that we love with a fraction of the carbs of a traditional version. The pastry is perfectly buttery and the filling simple and creamy. Serve on its own, with raspberries, crème fraîche or cream. Inulin is derived from chicory root and gives a caramelized glaze to the tart without having to use sugar.

Preheat the oven to 190°C/170°C fan/375°F/gas mark 5 and grease a 23cm (9in) fluted loose-bottomed tart tin with butter.

Mix the pastry ingredients together in a bowl with a metal spoon or spatula until well blended. Bring the mixture into a ball with your hands and transfer to a piece of baking parchment. Wrap it up and transfer to the freezer for 20 minutes.

Remove the pastry from the freezer and unwrap it, leaving the dough in the centre of the parchment. Put another piece of baking parchment on the top and roll out the pastry to a circle about 30cm (12in) wide and 5mm (¼in) thick. Peel off the top sheet of parchment and cut it into a circle just bigger than the tart tin and set aside. Pick up the piece of parchment with the pastry on it and turn it over on to the prepared tin. Carefully peel off the parchment and prick the pastry with a fork a few times to stop it rising.

Put the circle of baking parchment into the tin on top of the pastry and fill with rice or baking beans. Blind bake for 15 minutes.

Meanwhile, make the filling by mixing the lemon juice, eggs, honey or erythritol and double cream together in a bowl. Sieve the mixture into a jug and add the lemon zest.

Remove the parchment and beans from the pastry case and return it to the oven for a further 10–15 minutes until it is lightly golden brown. Set aside. Reduce the oven temperature to 150°C/130°C fan/300°F/gas mark 2.

Pour the lemon filling into the tart case, being careful not to spill the mixture. We find it easier to do this if the tart case is in the oven on a pulled-out rack. Bake for 20 minutes or until the filling is wobbly but just set.

Remove from the oven and leave to cool to room temperature. If you want a crunchy glaze, scatter the inulin evenly over the tart and use a cook's blowtorch to briefly scorch it all over. Once cool, keep in the fridge for a couple of days.

STRAWBERRY & VANILLA VERRINES

L

SERVES 6

For the strawberry jelly

3 gelatine leaves (I use Dr. Oetker)

350g (12oz) frozen or fresh strawberries, roughly chopped

1 tablespoon honey or 2 tablespoons powdered erythritol

1 teaspoon vanilla extract

For the vanilla cream

2 gelatine leaves

2 egg yolks

250ml (9fl oz) whole cow's or almond milk

½ vanilla pod or 2 teaspoons vanilla extract

1 tablespoon honey or 2 tablespoons powdered erythritol

75ml (2½fl oz) double cream

Per serving
with honey

17.6g net carbs, 2g fibre, 5.3g protein, 9g fat, 172kcal

with erythritol

6.5g net carbs, 1.2g fibre, 5g protein, 9g fat, 128kcal

We use fresh berries in summer and frozen strawberries in winter to make this decadent, diminutive dessert. Gelatine leaves can differ, so if you use another brand or use powdered gelatine, do read the packet instructions. You should be left with about 300ml (10fl oz) strained strawberry juice so you can follow the suggested ratio. As a natural alternative we have used honey for the jelly but dates for the vanilla cream. You can also make this in a square mould, cut it into squares once set and serve with fresh berries and either Greek yogurt or whipped cream.

Soak the gelatine leaves for the jelly in cold water. Put the strawberries, honey or erythritol and vanilla into a saucepan over a medium heat and bring to a gentle boil. You can do this with frozen berries, there is no need to defrost them. Cook for 5–7 minutes until softened.

Mash the strawberries smooth with a potato masher. Squeeze the liquid from the gelatine leaves and add them to the pan, then stir through until they disappear. Strain the mixture through a sieve into a jug, pushing as much pulp through as possible with a spatula or the back of a spoon, so you are only left with the pips to discard. Divide the strawberry jelly between 6 glasses and put into the fridge to set.

To make the vanilla cream, soak the gelatine leaves in cold water. Put the egg yolks, milk, vanilla and the honey or erythritol in a medium saucepan and whisk until completely smooth. Put the saucepan over a medium–high heat and bring to a gentle boil for about 2 minutes, whisking constantly. Remove from the heat. Squeeze out the water from the gelatine leaves and add them to the vanilla mixture. Whisk through until they disappear.

Pour the vanilla cream into a bowl through a sieve and set this bowl over another one full of iced water to cool. Whip the double cream to the consistency of thick yogurt. As soon as the vanilla cream is cool to touch (it will happen quickly, so don't let it set in the bowl), use a large spoon to fold in the whipped cream.

Check that the jelly is set enough to hold the cream, then divide the vanilla cream between the glasses. Return them to the fridge for at least 1 hour and up to 2 days before serving.

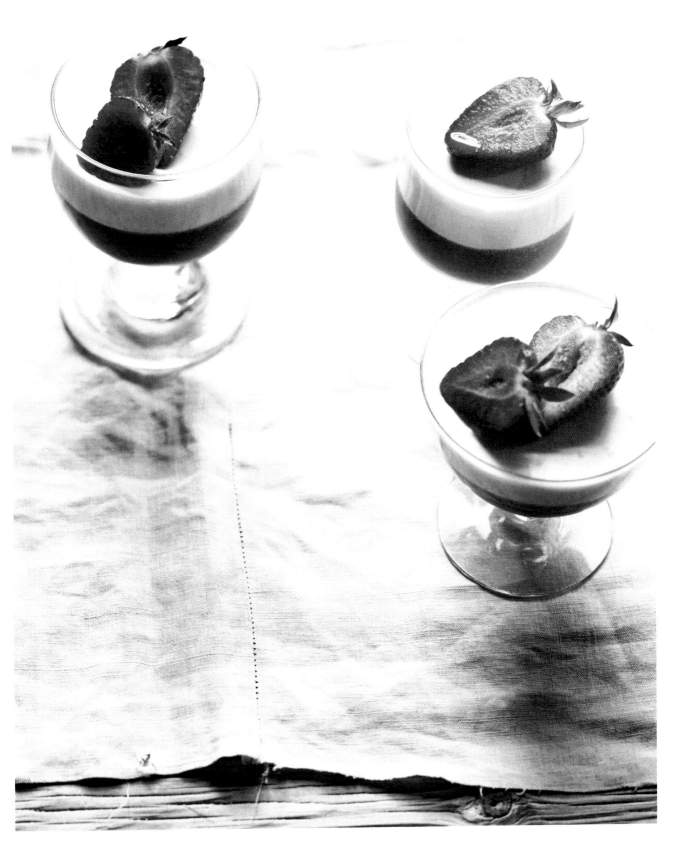

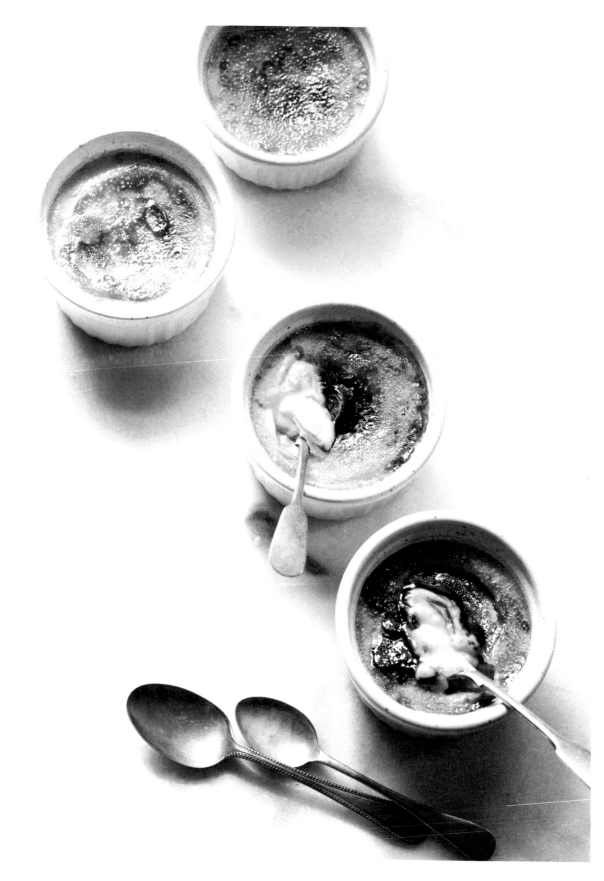

GINGER CRÈME BRÛLÉE

SERVES 6

90g (3¼oz) fresh ginger, peeled

450ml (16fl oz) double cream

2 teaspoons vanilla extract

6 egg yolks

4 tablespoons honey or 150g (5½oz) erythritol

6 teaspoons inulin powder (optional)

Per serving
with honey
15.9g net carbs, 2.8g fibre,
3.8g protein, 41.9g fat, 457kcal

with erythritol
4.3g net carbs, 2.8g fibre,
3.7g protein, 41.9g fat, 414kcal

Because Giancarlo is gluten intolerant, most of the options on a dessert menu are out of the question, but a crème brûlée is impossible for him to resist. However, we have now made one with erythritol or minimal honey so he can finally enjoy it again as a treat. It's still high in calories, so it really is a once-in-a-blue-moon occurrence. We love the flavour of ginger so have made this dessert quite punchy, but you can omit the ginger altogether if you prefer the simple taste of vanilla. The leftover egg whites can be frozen or used for the meringues on page 196. We have used inulin, an insoluble fibre from chicory root, to make the glaze, as it works like sugar, but you can leave this out if you wish. The erythritol does form a natural slightly crunchy topping, which is a pleasant contrast to the creamy brûlée.

Preheat the oven to 160°C/140°C fan/325°F/gas mark 3. Arrange 6 ramekins about 8 x 4cm (3¼ x 1½in) in a roasting tray. You can also use small tea or coffee cups instead.

Either grate the ginger or put it into a small food processor and blend to a purée. Add the ginger purée to a saucepan with the cream and vanilla. Put this over a medium–high heat and bring to the boil. Remove the pan from the heat and set aside.

Mix the egg yolks with the honey or erythritol in a mixing bowl with a whisk. Sieve the ginger cream on to the egg mixture and whisk together. Transfer the mixture to a jug and divide between the ramekins in the roasting tray.

Transfer the tray to the oven and pour cold water into the tray around the ramekins so that the water comes halfway up the sides. Close the oven and cook for 25 minutes or until just firm to the touch. You can put a knife in at the edge of a crème brûlée to check it is set around the edges. The centre should still be a little wobbly underneath the surface.

Remove from the oven and leave the brûlées to cool in the water. Once they are at room temperature, transfer to the fridge and leave for 6 hours or overnight.

If using the inulin, when you are about to serve, scatter 1 teaspoon of inulin evenly over each brûlée. Use a cook's blowtorch or a hot grill to brown the inulin; it will caramelize like sugar. Serve straight away.

Nutrient tables

These tables are to help familiarize you with carbohydrate levels of foods, together with fat, protein and fibre content. Each recipe in this book has the nutrient levels already calculated for you. Another source of info is an app or book such as *Carbs & Cals*. Please be aware that there is some discrepancy between different sources of nutrient info so try to choose one method for tracking and stick to it or things can get confusing!

PROTEIN FOODS – Meat

	Weight	calories	fat	carb	fibre	protein
Chicken, breast	120g	174	2	0	0	38
Chicken, thigh	120g	193	7	0	0	33
Turkey breast	120g	186	2	0	0	42
Turkey, dark meat	120g	213	8	0	0	35
Venison	120g	198	3	0	0	43
Duck	120g	234	12	0	0	30
Lamb leg	120g	290	16	0	0	36
Lamb shoulder	120g	282	16	0	0	34
Pork chop	120g	302	18	0	0	32
Pork scratchings	30g	182	14	0	0	14
Pork roast	120g	258	12	0	0	37
Sausages 97% meat (2)	117g	301	24	2	1	19
Bacon (2 rashers)	60g	172	13	0	0	14
Sirloin steak	200g	425	25	0	0	50
Roast beef	120g	293	15	0	0	39
Breaded chicken	120g	281	14	17	1	21

PROTEIN FOODS – Eggs & dairy

	Weight	calories	fat	carb	fibre	protein
Eggs (one)	54g	97	7	0	0	8
Full-fat Greek yogurt	100g	133	6	5	0	6
Low-fat fruit yogurt	100g	82	1	13	0	4
Cheddar	75g	311	26	0	0	19
Feta	75g	186	15	1	0	11
Roquefort	75g	280	25	0	0	14
Milk (full fat)	200ml	126	7	9	0	7
Milk (semi-skimmed)	200ml	94	3	9	0	7
Milk (skimmed)	200ml	70	1	9	0	7
Double cream	30ml	149	16	0	0	0

PROTEIN FOODS – Seafood

	Weight	calories	fat	carb	fibre	protein
Salmon	120g	245	15	0	0	28
Mackerel	120g	339	27	0	0	24
Prawns, peeled, frozen	120g	86	0.2	0	0	19
Sardines, canned	85g	187	12	0	0	20
Cod in breadcrumbs, baked	120g	242	14	12	1	17

PROTEIN – Vegetarian

	Weight	calories	fat	carb	fibre	protein
Puy lentils, half pack	125g	180	2	24	8	12
Chickpeas, half pack	115g	130	3	14	10	8

STARCHY FOODS – Veg

	Weight	calories	fat	carb	fibre	protein
Beetroot	100g	41	0	7	2	2
Butternut squash	100g	42	0	8	2	1
Carrots	100g	44	0	8	4	0
Celeriac	100g	26	0	2	4	1
Parsnip	100g	73	1	12	5	2
Potato	100g	75	0	17	2	2
Pumpkin	100g	15	0	2	1	1
Swede	100g	30	0	5	2	1
Sweet potato	100g	91	0	20	2	1
Sweetcorn	80g	55	2	6	3	2
Turnip	100g	30	0	5	2	1

STARCHY FOODS – Grains

	Weight	calories	fat	carb	fibre	protein
Brown bread (1 slice)	40g	86	1	15	2	4
Brown rice	50g	177	1	35	3	5
Chapatti	55g	186	7	24	3	5
Oats	35g	137	3	22	3	4
Pasta	75g	261	2	51	4	9
Quinoa	50g	160	3	26	4	7
Rye bread (1 slice)	72g	163	1	30	3	6
White bread (1 slice)	40g	89	1	17	1	4
White rice	50g	171	1	37	1	4

SUPERVEG

	Weight	calories	fat	carb	fibre	protein
Asparagus	80g	23	0	2	1	2
Aubergine	80g	16	0	2	2	1
Avocado, half	80g	158	16	2	3	2
Broccoli	80g	35	0	3	3	3
Brussel sprouts	80g	41	1	3	3	3
Cabbage	80g	25	0	4	2	1
Cauliflower	80g	33	0	6	1	2
Celery	80g	10	0	2	1	0
Courgettes	80g	18	0	1	2	1
Cucumber	80g	13	0	1	1	1
Fennel	80g	16	0	1	3	1
Garlic	10g	11	0	2	0	1
Green beans	80g	25	0	2	3	2
Kale	80g	33	1	1	3	3
Lettuce	60g	8	0	1	1	1
Leeks	80g	22	0	2	2	1
Mooli	80g	13	0	2	0	1
Mushrooms	80g	17	0	2	1	2
Olives	15g	17	2	0	1	0
Onions	50g	21	0	4	1	1
Peas	80g	62	1	8	4	4
Peppers	60g	16	0	3	1	0
Rocket	60g	13	0	0	1	2
Spinach	60g	11	0	0	1	2
Tomatoes	60g	13	0	2	1	0
Watercress	60g	17	1	0	2	2

FRUIT

	Weight	calories	fat	carb	fibre	protein
Apples	130g	56	0	13	1	0
Apricot	55g	17	0	4	1	1
Apricot, dried (4)	32g	81	0	16	7	2
Banana	130g	69	0	17	1	1
Blackberries	80g	20	0	4	3	1
Blueberries	80g	32	0	7	2	1
Cherries	100g	48	0	12	1	1
Dates (4)	30g	81	0	20	2	1
Grapefruit	114g	2	0	1	0	0
Honeydew melon	160g	45	0	11	2	2
Kiwi	55g	27	0	6	1	1
Mango	120g	68	0	17	5	1
Nectarine	140g	56	0	13	3	1
Orange	140g	38	0	8	1	1
Papaya	80g	29	0	7	2	0
Peach	140g	46	0	11	3	1
Pineapple	150g	75	0	15	3	0
Plum	110g	40	0	10	2	1
Pomegranate	80g	67	1	13	2	1
Raspberries	80g	20	0	4	2	1
Strawberries	140g	42	0	8	6	1
Sultanas	30g	83	0	21	1	1

OILS – Oil & fats

	Weight	calories	fat	carb	fibre	protein
Butter	10g	75	8	0	0	0
Coconut oil	10g	90	10	0	0	0
Olive oil	10g	90	10	0	0	0

OILS – Nuts & seeds

	Weight	calories	fat	carb	fibre	protein
Almonds	30g	185	16	2	5	6
Brazil nuts	30g	212	20	1	2	5
Cashews	30g	178	14	5	1	6
Coconut, desiccated	30g	196	19	2	6	2
Flaxseeds	30g	151	11	5	8	6
Hazelnuts	30g	204	19	2	3	5
Peanuts	30g	181	16	2	2	8
Pumpkin seeds	30g	170	14	5	2	8
Sesame seeds	30g	179	17	0	2	6
Sunflower seeds	30g	173	14	6	2	7
Walnuts	30g	213	21	1	2	5

INDEX

Resources

We use www.nutritics.com and www.cronometer.com for the nutritional analysis of the recipes.

Carbs & Cals produce carb and calorie counter books and apps.

Freestyle Libre makes instant glucose monitoring systems and can be found at www.freestylelibre.co.uk

The Public Health Collaboration (PHC) is a charity dedicated to informing and implementing healthy decisions for better public health. Find out more at www.phcuk.org

www.dietdoctor.com for a mass of well researched and evidence-based information on going low-carb and keto.

Giancarlo, Jenny and I were delighted to work with **Dr David Unwin** and **Dr Jen Unwin** on this project. Their knowledge, experience and help were invaluable. We wish it to be known that they have received no fee for their participation in this book. Instead, we made a donation to the Public Health Collaboration to further their work spreading the real food message.

Social media

Follow **Katie Caldesi** on social media @KatieCaldesi (Instagram and Twitter) or see our site www.thegoodkitchentable.com. Our restaurants and cookery schools are at www.caldesi.com or see Facebook under **thegoodkitchentable** or **Caldesi Italian Restaurants**.

Dr David Unwin tweets and can be contacted @lowcarbGP

Dr Jen Unwin, Clinical Psychologist, can be found on Twitter at @jen_unwin. For further information on carb addiction, see her book and her site at www.forkintheroad.co.uk

Jenny Phillips is on Twitter @jennynutrition and her website is www.inspirednutrition.co.uk

A huge thank you to…

Our publisher, **Joanna Copestick**.

Everyone who suggested and tested recipes with me for this book, including **Anne Hudson**, **the Soin family**, **Stefano Borella**, **Brian McLeod**.

Jonathan Hayden, our literary agent.

Vicky Orchard, editor.

Susan Bell, for the stunning photography.

Becks Wilkinson, for the beautiful food styling.

Hannah Wilkinson, for the prop styling.

Tina Smith Hobson, for the design of the book.

Emily Noto, for the production.

Our boys **Giorgio** and **Flavio**, for their help in shopping, cooking, tasting good (and bad!) recipes and constant washing and drying up.

OUR STORIES

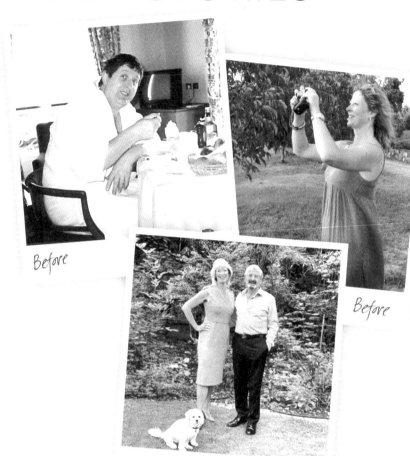

Before

Before

Before

After

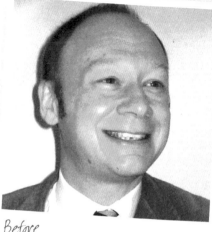

Before

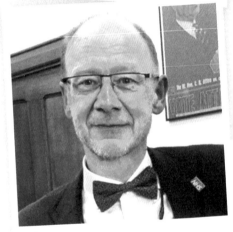

After

Katie & Giancarlo

Having followed a low-carb lifestyle for more than 10 years, we are convinced it is the only way to eat for us. It provides energy, nutrition and a positive mental attitude while giving us the freedom to enjoy the foods we love without feeling hungry. Giancarlo has lost over 4 stone and is in his 8th year of remission from type 2 diabetes. His joints are better, and he can exercise once more – we even bought him a bicycle for his 69th birthday!

Dr David Unwin

As you can see, cutting the carbs caused me to lose about 2 stone in weight, so my waist now is the same as when I was half my current age! More important to me are the improvements in my blood pressure. Also I have more energy, needing 90 minutes less sleep a day and I can still jog 5 miles several times a week. For me, giving up table sugar, bread, biscuits and potatoes has been well worth it!